MY MINI
MIDWIFE

MY MINI MIDWIFE

Vie Books is an imprint of Summersdale Publishers Ltd

Summersdale Publishers Ltd
46 West Street
Chichester
West Sussex
PO19 1RP
UK

www.summersdale.com

Printed and bound by CPI Group (UK) Ltd, Croydon, CR0 4YY

ISBN: 978-1-84953-516-8

Substantial discounts on bulk quantities of Summersdale books are available to corporations, professional associations and other organisations. For details contact Nicky Douglas by telephone: +44 (0) 1243 756902, fax: +44 (0) 1243 786300 or email: nicky@summersdale.com.

DISCLAIMER
My Mini Midwife is intended for use as a guide only. It is not to be used in place of a consultation with your maternity healthcare professional.

Although all maternity care practices are safe and appropriate to meet the needs of pregnant women, newborns and new parents, services offered at maternity units can vary widely. So you may find that the care you receive and the options you are offered are different to those available elsewhere.

Everything
you need to know
about pregnancy
and birth

MY MINI
MIDWIFE

DENYSE KIRKBY

ABOUT THE AUTHOR

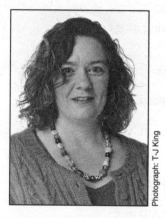

Photograph: T-J King

Denyse Kirkby is a registered midwife (RM), registered midwifery teacher (RMT), Higher Education Academy (HEA) fellow and United Kingdom Public Health Register (UKPHR) registered public health practitioner (PHP).

She finished her three-year midwifery training in 1997 and since then has enjoyed the privilege of working as a registered midwife in delivery, antenatal and postnatal suites in a number of different hospitals, as well as working as a community midwife and a specialist antenatal and newborn screening midwife. In 2008 Denyse decided that she wanted to share her knowledge and help shape the working practices of future midwives, and so began her training to become a registered midwifery teacher. One thing led to another and she now has three qualifications: midwifery, midwifery teaching and public health practitioner.

She lives in the south of England in a home otherwise filled with males – husband, boys and pets: she writes books for adults and children to escape the testosterone. Using the pseudonym D. J. Kirkby she wrote *Without Alice*, *My Dream of You* and *Special Deliveries: Life Changing Moments* and wrote the Portal Series for children as Dee Kirkby. In her spare time she enjoys family time, reading, baking and running

Find out more about D. J. Kirkby on her websites:

- Writing for adults: **www.djkirkby.co.uk**

- Writing for children: **www.deekirkby.co.uk**

Follow D. J. Kirkby on Twitter:

www.twitter.com/djkirkby

Find D. J. Kirkby on Facebook:

https://www.facebook.com/DeeJKirkby

PREFACE

You may be planning your pregnancy or you may be already pregnant and you probably have a lot of questions. Whether this is your first pregnancy or your fourth, each one is different and *My Mini Midwife* is designed to help you answer those questions. You'll be going through physical and emotional changes during this exciting and unique time of your life. You may have questions about what is 'normal', or why your body is doing things at certain stages.

My Mini Midwife is designed to suit your needs and those of everyone to whom your pregnancy is important. It is designed to be practical in nature: you can use it to find clear answers to questions as and when they arise, dip into it for guidance as to what you should do in certain situations, or read it from cover to cover. Tucked away inside *My Mini Midwife* you will find advice on planning your pregnancy and on taking control of and making the most of your pregnancy, labour and birth, and more. With your copy of this book as a reference and in partnership with your real-life midwife, general practitioner (GP) and other healthcare professionals such as an obstetrician or other specialist, you will be able to make the most of this memorable time in your life. If you would like to read the most up-to-date guidance, there is a section for this on my website: **www.djkirkby.co.uk/my-mini-midwife**.

The anecdotes in *My Mini Midwife* have been fictionalised in order to maintain the anonymity of those I have cared for and worked with throughout the years. Therefore any resemblance to persons living or dead is entirely coincidental.

CONTENTS

THE COUNTDOWN STARTS HERE

At least twelve months before you begin trying to conceive a baby it's advisable to try to get into the best possible shape and adopt a healthy lifestyle. Ideally you should aim to stop smoking and drink alcohol in moderation only – by this I mean no more than two units in a week, with at least a day off before you drink alcohol again. The current guidance to women is to avoid alcohol while trying to conceive and while pregnant. If you have tried, and failed, to stop smoking in the past please don't be disheartened and do try again. One of these times it will work!

During your countdown phase you should also make an appointment to see your GP, so that you can tell him/her that you are planning to become pregnant. Make a list of things to discuss with your GP, which should include:

- Any prescribed medications you currently take and if they are suitable for pregnancy and breastfeeding (also inform your GP if you are using any recreational drugs because these will have an effect on you, your baby and how your body copes with your pregnancy; your doctor will keep this information confidential).

- When to stop using a hormonal contraceptive and which other contraception method you should use, and for how long.

- When you should have your next cervical smear test.

- If all your immunisations are up-to-date.

- If you need any other screening for infections like chlamydia or syphilis (which can take a long time to show any symptoms), or for illnesses such as diabetes.

- Is your weight within a healthy range to encourage conception and/or sustain a pregnancy?

- Do you need genetic screening for such diseases as cystic fibrosis, sickle cell and thalassaemia? This will be offered by your midwife if you fit the screening criteria (for example, if you have a family history of these disorders), but the earlier you can have these tests, the better.

- Many women who do not plan their pregnancies have no knowledge of the fact that they are pregnant for the first few weeks, and yet this is the time when many fetal problems related to lifestyle or chronic diseases such as diabetes are thought to occur.

- There are many screening tests which your GP or midwife may want to do when you are planning a pregnancy, or are in early pregnancy. These tests range from taking blood, checking your blood pressure and measuring your height and weight to scans of your baby and more. Please see the 'Screening and Diagnostic Tests' chapter in this book for further information. You are expected to give consent for these screening tests, so don't be afraid to ask for more information or a leaflet to take away and read if you need it before agreeing to have the test.

Some areas offer midwifery- or practice nurse-led pre-conception clinics where you can discuss the issues listed above and more, so ask at your GP surgery if this is an option for you.

THE TWELVE-MONTH PREGNANCY

So you've decided you want to have a baby? Congratulations, you have taken the first step towards becoming a parent. Your body is going to be your baby's home for the duration of your pregnancy and you have recognised the need to make it the best you can offer to your unborn child. Everyone should view pregnancy as lasting at least twelve months (with three months falling into the period before you become pregnant), meaning pre-conception care is especially important for everyone, but particularly if you have medical problems or pre-existing conditions. The better prepared you are, the better you will cope with this major life change.

Adopt a healthier lifestyle

Try to have a parenting partnership in which you encourage each other to adopt similarly healthy lifestyles at least twelve months before you begin trying to conceive your baby.

Exercise

Start or continue to exercise daily for as long as you can manage comfortably. I strongly recommend at least thirty minutes of daily gentle exercise, such as walking or swimming in a warm pool, as a minimum: if you can manage more than this, then do so. Exercise helps your body do everything more efficiently. When you exercise, your body processes medications more effectively and also digests food better (helping you to maintain a healthy weight), your sleep patterns are more restorative and your mood is elevated in comparison to when your body receives no exercise.

Folic acid and vitamins

When you stop using your hormonal contraceptive you should begin taking 400 micrograms of folic acid (0.4 mg) each day, even though you won't be trying to conceive straight away. Your body will benefit from some time to clear any remaining hormones from your system. The folic acid won't do you any harm, and taking it before you become pregnant will give you time to make it into a habit. Folic acid helps prevent some structural problems in babies, particularly ones of the brain and spinal cord (these are also known as neural tube defects). You should also eat foods which are rich in folic acid, such as green leafy vegetables, nuts, cooked dried beans, citrus fruits, avocado, raspberries and raw mushrooms. If you take a vitamin supplement, make sure that it is clearly indicated on the packaging that is suitable for pregnancy, as certain vitamins are not safe to take in pregnancy. If you are not certain if the vitamin supplement of your choosing is safe, then you can ask any chemist or your GP, practice nurse or midwife.

If you drink herbal teas check they are safe during pregnancy. The same goes for any essential perfume oils you may use, as well as certain bath products that may contain them. Oils such as rose and clary sage are not safe to use during pregnancy, so be sure to ask for advice before buying them. During my career I have seen women use many different types of natural remedies.

These often made me feel a bit nervous, as most people don't seem to realise that they aren't just nice-smelling products; these oils, tinctures, tablets and teas often contain properties of a medicinal nature.

One woman I cared for was extremely fond of herbal treatments and had a veritable cornucopia in her home from which she mixed her own herbal teas, bath products and remedies for various minor ailments. She had several certificates from courses she had attended in order to learn how to use herbs as medicine and had great faith in her ability to treat any ailment she or her husband had. I made sure that she knew that her local hospital had strict policies about the use of certain oils, and that as a midwife without specialist training in aromatherapy I would not be able to participate or advise in this area of labour care. Midwives are not legally allowed to advise and support women in using alternative therapies unless we have undertaken specialised training, and this is why we advise against the use of essential oils unless you have the necessary specialist support.

Essential fatty acids

Increase your intake of essential fatty acids to help maximise fertility. They are also good for the development of your baby's nervous system and brain and can be found in foods which contain the oils omega-3, -6 and -9.

- Omega-3 is found in oily fish, such as mackerel, and in green leafy vegetables.

- Omega-6 is found in most vegetable cooking oils, but not in olive oil.

- Omega-9 is found in olive oil.

Protein

Protein-rich food is an essential part of our diet and can be found in foods such as eggs, meat, pulses and grains such as quinoa. Eat no more than a palm-sized amount of protein with each meal in order to keep your plate of food and diet balanced. Every plate of food should be divided into quarters, with two quarters used for vegetables and fruit, one quarter pasta, rice or potatoes and the other quarter reserved for your protein such as meat, fish, poultry or a substitute such as tofu or Quorn.

Calcium

This helps strengthen bones and helps your body absorb vitamin D. Calcium is found in foods such as cheese, yogurt, milk, ice cream, kale, Swiss chard, broccoli, tofu and tinned salmon or sardines.

Vitamin D

This is important in helping your body absorb and use calcium as well as other substances needed for the formation of healthy bones and teeth. The best food source for vitamin D is oily fish such as salmon, sardines, pilchards and trout, but it is also found in good amounts in dairy products, egg yolks and vitamin D-fortified spreads and breakfast cereals. Vitamin D is found in small amounts in mushrooms and dark leafy greens (such as kale and spinach).

- Try to eat foods in a variety of colours at each meal to ensure that your diet is balanced. For example, a dish of (free-range) meat or fresh fish, red, green and yellow roasted peppers (try coating them in pesto sauce before popping them under the grill), carrots and broccoli and some potatoes or rice creates a meal containing many vitamins and minerals which are vital for health.

- Avoid unpasteurised products during pregnancy (the labelling should say if they are unpasteurised, but don't be afraid to ask if you can't see it written on the label).

For mon

Maximise sperm count and mobility by wearing loose underwear such as boxers instead of close-fitting pants, and by eating regular portions of fish, eggs, mushrooms, oysters, pumpkin seeds and other zinc-rich foods. Smoking and alcohol have been found to reduce sperm counts and to increase the production of damaged sperm.

Odds and ends

Visit your dentist early on in your twelve-month pregnancy, preferably before you become pregnant, in order to complete any dental work you may require and to gain advice about what changes pregnancy may cause to your teeth and gums. Dentists will be reluctant to carry out any dental work on pregnant woman. You may notice that your gums swell or bleed during pregnancy due to the hormonal changes. This is quite normal and usual gum health should return soon after the birth of your baby. Maintaining good oral hygiene as well as seeing a dental hygienist regularly can help with this.

If you haven't managed to stop smoking yet, you (and your partner) should do so at least four months before you begin trying to get pregnant, as well as avoiding alcohol and any unnecessary drugs.

Finally, and perhaps most important of all, enjoy and cherish the company of your partner during this exciting time in your lives.

Health fact

It is thought that passive smoking can harm your unborn baby almost as much as if you were the one doing the smoking, so try to avoid situations where you will be exposing yourself and your unborn baby to cigarette smoke.

CONCEPTION AND MOVING FORWARD

Attempting conception

This is by far one of the most intricate and complex functions your body will ever perform, and you are likely to be blissfully unaware that it has done so flawlessly. The very first step in this amazing process is when an egg cell from the woman is fertilised by a sperm cell from a man. Sounds simple, but it is far from it. In order for conception to occur, the egg and sperm cells must first be in the same place at the same time.

There are several ways this can happen: in a heterosexual relationship try to make love a few times a week. (Sperm will usually live for three to five days inside a woman's body, so don't worry if you make love less often.) Remember, this is supposed to be an exciting and celebratory time in your lives, so vary the positions you use and the times of day you try, and above all, avoid letting it become a mechanical procedure you repeat with military precision.

If you are in a female same-sex relationship then you must first decide which of you will become pregnant. There are a few ways to obtain sperm, some more safe and advisable than others. There are services which match lesbian couples with vetted sperm donors, although the two parties never meet. The sperm donation is made through one of a network of clinics and then despatched to the recipients so they can carry out insemination at home. However, there are other sperm donor services available. Or you might decide to do it privately, using a male acquaintance or friend as donor. I would advise caution with both of these options. Do not put yourself in a situation where your safety may be compromised; the same goes for protecting your health. You need to be able to assure yourself that the sperm is donated from someone who has had a very recent sexual health screen and, ideally, always has protected intercourse. Remember, his sperm is going into your body, which is the same as if you were having unprotected sex with him, so you are at risk of any sexually transmitted infection he may have, such as chlamydia, hepatitis B and C or HIV. There are also legal aspects to consider, such as whether he will have any contact with the child, and so on. It would be wise to consult with a solicitor on this matter.

If you are in a male same-sex relationship then surrogacy may be an option you wish to consider. Surrogacy enables a male couple to father a child without the mother being involved in the baby's upbringing. The 'traditional' method involves a surrogate mother using her own eggs and being inseminated with the sperm of the father. The second option is known as gestational surrogacy, involving one woman serving as the egg donor and another woman being pregnant with the baby. The eggs are fertilised with the sperm artificially, and the resultant embryo is transferred to the gestational surrogate (the one who gets pregnant and gives birth). As above, there are also legal aspects to consider, such as whether the mother will have any contact with the child. Again, it would be wise to consult with a solicitor on this matter.

Make lovemaking enjoyable

Many people who are actively trying to get pregnant find the intent of it all somewhat discomfiting, so it is important that you both work on finding out what is most comfortable and enjoyable for you. Take as much time as you want to pamper and prepare yourself. Be aware that some medications can decrease your libido, as can work-related stress. You may find that one of the many lubricants designed to enhance enjoyment will help. Some lubricants warm whichever part of the body you choose to put them on, so try different areas such as your nipples, as well as the more obvious ones. They are easily available from most pharmacies and some supermarkets, in the family planning section.

Choose a position that is the most comfortable for you. If you can, try to make love until you reach orgasm, as this makes your cervix dip into the pool of sperm and there is some thought that this creates a bit of a vacuum to help move the sperm in the right direction. There are no hard-and-fast rules except one: 'If you don't enjoy it, don't do it!'

Contrary to popular belief, a bath or shower after lovemaking will not wash the sperm away; enough will stay inside to give conception a good chance. It only takes one to get to the egg to do the job; all the rest of the sperm are superfluous (and responsible for non-identical twins).

Do I have fertility problems?

It is perfectly normal to take up to a year or longer to get pregnant, so just try to relax and enjoy this stage of your lives. One useful tip for men is to avoid tight underwear during this time to allow the testicles to stay away from the body, providing a beneficial, cooler environment for the sperm.

For women, conditions such as endometriosis (in moderate to severe cases) can reduce fertility. Mild endometriosis is not thought to be associated with reduced fertility. If you have endometriosis you can discuss what options are available to you with your GP or specialist when planning your pregnancy. Once pregnant, the discomfort and pain caused by endometriosis can lessen and for some disappears for the duration of the pregnancy.

Every pregnancy carries a risk of sexually transmitted infections (because you've had unprotected sex), both for you and your unborn child, so please make sure that you are certain that both you and your partner (and any third party involved in conception) are free of infections. Your GP or local sexual health clinic will be able to advise you further on this.

Conception completed

OK, so you've managed to conceive, now what happens? Well, you will likely carry on for a while unaware this miracle has occurred, but if this is a planned pregnancy you will be no doubt wondering if you've managed to accomplish it. The soonest you will know for certain will be around the time of your next expected menstrual period, though some pregnancy tests can now detect a pregnancy slightly earlier.

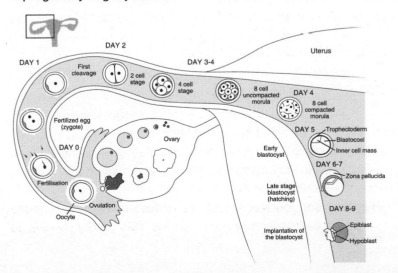

While you are waiting for the moment of truth, your body will be hard at work. The fertilised cell is floating down the fallopian tube towards the uterus (womb) and dividing itself into two cells: those two divide into four and so on for the following week. This is the time an ectopic pregnancy can occur: the growing cluster of cells decides to attach itself to the fallopian tube instead of the uterus. An ectopic pregnancy can develop into a life-threatening condition, so if you think you are showing any signs of an ectopic pregnancy contact your GP or the gynaecology department at your nearest hospital straight away.

Symptoms of an ectopic pregnancy can include one or many of the following:

- Sharp, stabbing pain in the lower back, or side-upper abdomen

- Pelvic heaviness or discomfort that occurs intermittently, consistently or when you are coughing or having a bowel movement

- One-sided pain in your pelvic or abdominal region

- Shoulder pain, particularly when you lie down (this can be a sign of blood in your abdomen)

- Sudden onset, severe and/or persistent pain

- Cramping that is more severe than your normal period cramps

- Nausea and vomiting (more extreme than that which you may already be feeling with your pregnancy)

- Clammy skin

- Racing, weak pulse

- Pale or ashen complexion

- Rapid drop in blood pressure (which will make you feel faint)

- Loss of mental alertness, or confusion

- A feeling of impending doom or an overwhelming feeling that something is seriously wrong in your body.

If the cluster of cells adopts the usual position of waiting until it reaches the uterus, then there is plenty of room for it to settle down and continue to grow. Now it really gets clever, as part of this cluster of cells carries on growing into an embryo which will in turn grow into your fetus (once born, the fetus becomes a baby, so I will refer to it as 'your baby' for the rest of this book), and the other part of the cluster of cells begin to form the placenta. The placenta connects with your bloodstream to obtain nourishment and oxygen. The placenta also produces hormones which stop you from having your period so that your pregnancy can continue; if all of this doesn't happen then your pregnancy would most likely be shed with the lining of the uterus (your menstrual period).

Odds and ends

Now that you have begun trying to conceive and are aware that you won't know you are pregnant for up to three weeks, there are some precautions you need to take:

- Try to reduce any possible exposure to hazardous fumes if you work in an environment where you may be exposed. If you do work in such an environment, then your health and safety department should have already made you aware of this, but if you are not sure then don't hesitate to ask them.

- Reduce your risk of eating foods containing the bacteria listeria by avoiding unpasteurised foods such as soft cheeses, raw milk, soft ice creams, pâté, raw meat, unwashed raw vegetables, smoked mussels, raw fish such as sushi and raw shellfish such as oysters. I would advise you to always read the food packaging to help avoid unpasteurised foods. Listeria can grow at very low temperatures, which is why it is important to cook foods at the temperature and for the length of time recommended on the packaging or in any recipe you may be following. If eating barbecued food, ensure it has been cooked slowly and thoroughly.

Health facts

Fish is an excellent source of nourishment at this time, but certain fish (sea perch, catfish, shark, bluefin tuna and marlin) are thought to be high in mercury levels and should be avoided. If you eat fish, you should try to have it at least twice a week to benefit from the omega-3 oils, and if you are vegetarian you should increase your dairy product intake and eat more pulses to ensure you are meeting your altered nutritional needs.

Avoid contact with pet litter (or wear gloves if you cannot avoid this) in order to reduce the chance of you coming into contact with toxoplasmosis, which can be found in animal faeces.

Be money wise

It is always the right time to begin saving money, even if it is just a few pence per day. Save it up during the week, and ideally make a monthly (or more frequent) deposit into a high-interest savings account.

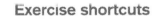

Exercise shortcuts

Walk whenever possible instead of taking the car. For example, you could walk to the shops when you only need to buy a few things, carpool or only drive or take public transport part of the way and then walk the rest. Your health will benefit and you will save the money you would have spent on petrol or the bus fare.

EARLY PREGNANCY

You are pregnant!

Well done! May I be the first – well OK, maybe the second or third – person to congratulate you on your success. I hope you had some fun getting to this stage. By this stage (about 5 weeks) I expect you will have already done a pregnancy test if you were planning on becoming pregnant. The tests are so sensitive now that they can detect your pregnancy as early as the first day of your missed period, although the indicator line may only show up as very faint: but faint or not, if it is there then so is your baby! From now until the end of week 10 your baby will make its presence known in a variety of ways: by changing the way things taste and smell, rewiring your emotions enough to make you want to weep at adverts for toilet roll and, for some, making even waking up a more tiring experience than usual. Sorry to have to be the one to break this to you, but you have just jumped onto the pregnancy roller coaster.

What you can do to make pregnancy symptoms easier to cope with

Stress

Keep your stress levels as low as possible. Have warm baths and try listening to relaxation tracks. Guided mental imagery (thinking of scenes, activities or places that make you happy) and progressive muscle relaxation (start at one end of your body, and imagine your muscles are relaxing one by one as you slowly work your way to the other end of your body) really do work and give you an excuse for lounging in the bath.

Exercise

By about week six your body will have increased your blood volume by about 50 per cent, and it is more important than ever that you keep as mobile as possible in order to help your body smoothly circulate this increased blood flow and to prevent blood clots. At risk of contradicting myself, I am also advising that you rest when you need to: your body is working extremely hard and you need to try and have short naps during the day, if possible. Even just ten minutes of sitting in a quiet place will help your body rest and relax.

Fatigue

It is perfectly normal during the first few months of pregnancy to feel completely drained of energy, and this is a symptom that has no cure except sleep. Naps help because little and often is better than none. If you need to go to bed at 4 p.m. to feel rested, then do so; you won't be any good to anyone if you wear yourself out completely. Avoid caffeine and other stimulants because they won't make you feel more awake and, as caffeine can cross the placental barrier, they are unsafe for your pregnancy in moderate to large doses. A little bit of caffeine in chocolate, for example, is an acceptable amount a few times a week and dark chocolate contains iron, which is good for you. Tea, hot chocolate and coffee are higher in caffeine and you should have no more than four cups per day, though most women will find themselves unable to tolerate the taste of coffee or tea during pregnancy.

Nausea

This is a very common side effect of pregnancy and most women have to endure nausea for at least a few weeks, with the majority of women complaining of nausea for the first few months and the occasional woman suffering for her entire pregnancy. Try to eat several small meals a day to ease the strain on your stomach, and if you are struggling to eat anything at all then try cubes of frozen crushed fruit. These also make nourishing mini-snacks.

Motion-sickness bands work well to ease the nausea and you can buy them without prescription at any major chemist. Ginger also helps and can be found in ginger snaps, ginger beer and tea, or in capsule form. If you feel so ill that you can't bear the thought of swallowing anything, try sprinkling a few drops of ginger essential oil on a warm flannel and inhaling the vapour or washing with ginger soap. Drink plenty of fluids because dehydration will make your nausea worse.

Cravings

These can start at any time during the pregnancy or not at all: simply eat what you crave, within moderation. Craving non-nutritional substances such as coal, the heads of matches, paper, ice, etc., to name but a few, is known as 'pica' rather than cravings, and if you experience this urge please discuss it with your midwife or doctor as some non-nutritional substances are harmful to your baby as well as yourself.

Mood swings (also known as the pregnancy roller coaster)

Mostly to blame for this somewhat bewildering sensation is the fact that your endocrine glands have put their feet on the accelerator pedal (in terms of hormone production) and are now in overdrive, without having given you time to even put on your seatbelt, and your placenta is about to do exactly the same. So yes, you do have an excuse for weeping copiously when your favourite houseplant dies. It is worth keeping in mind that if you suffered from low moods and depressions before pregnancy then you are more at risk of depression during and after pregnancy. If you or your partner are at all concerned, then talk to your midwife or doctor about what help is available, and do it sooner rather than later.

Libido

Early pregnancy, with its constant tiredness, nausea and mood swings, can make sex the furthest thing from your mind. However, for some women the increased blood flow to breasts and genitals can cause an increased sexual arousal and desire for sex. There is no right or wrong way to feel, and whichever way you do feel is likely to change as your pregnancy continues. Just to reassure you, penetrative sex is not linked with an increase in risk of miscarriage.

Don't forget your partner

While you are pregnant, your partner is going through changes, too. They will be going through changes, anxieties, fears, doubts and surges of joy – just like you!

Try to include your partner in the pregnancy as much as possible. This can be one of the closest emotional times in your relationship, so take the opportunity to discuss your expectations and fears. Make your partner a part of your daily exercises – for example, by going on evening walks or swims together. Bring your partner along to your antenatal appointments and encourage them to ask all the questions they have about the pregnancy. Also, try to maintain your physical intimacy, including sexual intercourse. If intercourse becomes uncomfortable, or it is recommended that you stop for medical reasons, try to find other ways to express your physical love. Go to birthing classes together, if they are offered at a suitable time in your area. As always, communication is an important aspect and it is worth remembering that your partner may feel left out and not really a part of things once you are pregnant. Your partner won't be able to experience the same changes you are going through at the same level as you, won't feel your baby moving until much later than you do and also may worry about how your baby will affect your ability to spend loving time together as a couple. Talk about the fears, concerns and delights both of you are experiencing.

Other children

If this isn't your first child, then you should consider when and how you give your other children advance notice about the new baby. Depending on the age of the child this may be a good time to tell them some of the key points about how babies are made and where babies come from, and there are many good picture books in your local libraries which will help you do this. Borrow or buy books and sit down with your child to read them together. Try not to take any concerns they may have lightly. It is common for siblings to feel they may get left out, or to have questions and worries about their position in the family. They need to be reassured before and after the birth that they are still loved. Tell them the truth about what being a big sibling is going to be like: that babies are a lot of fun and sometimes a lot of trouble, too. If you can prepare your child for the reality of having a new baby in the house then there will be less room for fear and resentment. It may help to ask your child how they feel about the baby before and after the birth. Listen to their answers and talk about them, but don't dismiss their anxieties by saying things like 'That's silly' or 'You shouldn't feel that way', because children usually have very mixed feelings about a new baby. Try including them in the pregnancy by letting them help with buying baby clothes and equipment and planning for the baby's arrival. Try not to be shy about your changing body. Let them see how it is making room for your growing baby.

A means to an end

I hope this hasn't seemed all doom and gloom. Although early pregnancy is sometimes a struggle, it is a struggle with a purpose. You are going through this while doing one of the most important jobs of your life: growing your baby. The symptoms won't last for ever: in fact, by week 11 or 12 you will begin feeling more like your old self, as your body begins to adjust to these changes.

Health fact

Folic acid helps your baby to grow strong bones and helps to prevent spina bifida. Folic acid can be found in many types of food, but is easily destroyed by cooking, so eat raw (and washed) lettuce and leafy green vegetables, cabbage, mushrooms, oranges and wholemeal bread.

Be money wise

Talk to your friends and relatives to find out what equipment and clothes they needed. They may have items their baby no longer needs which can be passed on to you, but if not, then look for baby and maternity clothes in charity shops. You will save money and help others at the same time. Additionally, parenting organisations host sales of clothes and equipment, so look on websites of such organisations as your local council, the NCT, BabyCentre or Netmums local online message boards, Facebook 'for sale' groups and so on for details of sales near you. Do not buy mattresses or car seats second-hand, as faults and hazards associated with these second-hand items are often invisible.

Exercise shortcuts

Many areas now offer organised healthy walks, so join one of these groups to increase your fitness and lower your stress levels.

Did you know?

Some maternity services now offer 'Early Bird' classes, which support you through making decisions about early-pregnancy screening and testing by offering you plenty of information. It is also an opportunity to meet others who are at the same stage of pregnancy.

SCREENING AND DIAGNOSTIC TESTS

Is my baby OK?

This question is likely to cross every expectant parent's mind at least once during the pregnancy. For those with pre-existing medical conditions, this worry can be magnified out of all proportion. However, there are many reassurances that pregnancy screening and diagnostic testing can provide, although there are also some questions that can never be completely answered until after your baby is born. The screening and tests described below should be offered to you and your partner as options. It is your choice whether or not to have them.

Routine blood screening and testing

Your blood is checked at the beginning of your pregnancy in order to get baseline levels with which to keep an eye on your overall health during your pregnancy, when some of the tests are repeated. New tests may be done, if necessary, to test for disorders of pregnancy that can occur in some women. A full-blood count is done to check levels of red (oxygen and iron-carrying) and white (infection-fighting) blood cells early on and part way through your pregnancy as routine, and more frequently if needed. Your blood is also checked for atypical antibodies; this test is discussed in more detail in the 'Less Common Changes and Complications during Pregnancy' chapter. Information from early-pregnancy blood testing also provides the necessary information needed to complete the first trimester screening of your baby (see later in this chapter for more on this test). Depending upon what your 'Family Origin Questionnaire' answers indicate, you may also be offered testing for sickle cell or thalassaemia.

Routine infectious diseases screening and testing

Numerous infectious diseases are routinely tested for during your pregnancy. These tests are not dependent on your history or lifestyle: they are simply offered to all women because the benefits of early diagnosis outweigh the cost of universal testing. HIV, syphilis, rubella and hepatitis B are tested for by taking blood, and chlamydia is tested for by using a urine sample. It is highly recommended that you undergo this testing because all of these diseases can show no symptoms for many years, and many of them are easily treated. Hepatitis C and Group B streptococcus (more information can be found on page 81) are not tested for routinely, but may be offered depending on your history or lifestyle.

Other screening options

These will give you a risk result reflecting the likelihood of your baby having certain genetic or structural disorders. They are usually calculated using a risk assessment form, scan or blood test or through a combination of all three, and do not directly carry a risk to you or your baby's health.

Ultrasound screening

An ultrasound in early pregnancy (around 11 weeks) can determine whether or not you are carrying multiple babies. Unlike X-rays, ultrasound uses sound waves to produce a video 'picture' of your baby inside your uterus. This picture is generated from an instrument, called a probe, that is placed either on your abdomen or in your vagina. Some women may find the full bladder required for a good scan at this stage of pregnancy incredibly uncomfortable. When you empty your bladder after the scan, the sudden release of fluid from your tense muscles may cause you to feel quite faint, so it would be sensible to ask your partner to come in the toilet with you. The hospital or scanning facility should have a toilet cubicle able to accommodate you both.

Ultrasound can be used to detect a problem or monitor a condition in your baby during pregnancy. From week 11 to week 13 (and up to six days after this), a nuchal translucency scan can be done to check for risk of chromosomal abnormalities such as Down's, Edward's and Patau's syndromes and is often combined with blood tests taken just before the scan. Your stage of pregnancy will be estimated from the first day of your last period, and then this will be confirmed at the beginning of your nuchal translucency scan in order to make sure your pregnancy is at the right stage for this screening to be done accurately. Your overall risk will be calculated from the results of both the scan and the blood tests. This is not a diagnostic test (i.e. one capable of giving a 'yes' or 'no' answer), but a form of screening which gives you a risk factor for these disorders. If your baby is considered to be at increased risk then an appointment will be made for you to discuss what options are available to you, including diagnostic testing.

If you are between four and six months pregnant and your baby is positioned correctly, a scan should be able to determine the sex of your baby, although some hospitals have a policy of not reporting on this, so you may need to pay privately to find out whether you are having a boy or a girl. If necessary, a scan can also be used to track the baby's growth, locate the placenta, determine how much fluid is around the baby, and detect some types of birth defects, such as ones involving the heart valves or kidneys. A full bladder is not required for a scan at this stage.

For more details about any of the screening and diagnostic tests in this book please visit: **www.djkirkby.co.uk/my-mini-midwife**, where you will find links to the most up-to-date information available.

Health fact

Caffeine crosses the placenta and may be harmful to your baby in large doses. A maximum of four cups of coffee, tea or cans of cola is considered to be within safe limits. If you would like more than that, then consider switching to caffeine-free versions.

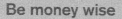

Be money wise

If receiving care from an independent midwife and/ or doula interests you, then make an appointment to speak to one or both as soon as possible, because you will need to pay for this care. Most will offer a payment plan to help you spread the cost. To find an independent midwife near you, go to the Independent Midwives UK website (www.independentmidwives. org.uk) *and enter your postcode, and to find your nearest doula, go to the Doula UK website* (doula.org. uk) *and enter your postcode.*

Exercise shortcuts

When you are sitting down or standing still (for example, when washing your hands or doing the dishes), tighten your buttocks or the muscle you use to urinate, hold for a count of twenty and then relax. This is a good exercise for working your pelvic floor muscles. These exercises should be done regularly to help prevent the incontinence that may occur later in life, and after birth these exercises will increase the flow of blood to your pelvic floor, which will help you heal and tighten up.

Did you know?

When you travel, and in particular if travelling when pregnant, you should take regular rest breaks (including a short walk) to improve your circulation and to stretch and loosen your body.

Screening and Diagnostic Tests

If you choose to have first trimester screening done, then three or four hormone levels (the number varies between hospitals) will be measured in your blood and the results are combined with information on your age, weight, whether you are a smoker, your ethnicity, your baby's neural tube measurement and the stage of pregnancy. A computer program then works out the risk of your baby having Down's syndrome, Patau's syndrome, Edward's syndrome or spina bifida. For more details about any of the screening and diagnostic tests in this book please visit **www.djkirkby.co.uk/my-mini-midwife**, where you will find links to the most up-to-date information available. If you have further questions about these conditions then your midwife will be happy to answer them for you.

Further testing, such as detailed ultrasound and/or amniocentesis, may be required with an increased-risk result. This additional test is offered in order to be able to give you more definitive answers, but you are not obligated to undergo this additional testing if you don't want to.

Risk results and what happens next

If you have been identified as being at increased risk of carrying a baby with a health complication you will be offered an appointment to discuss your options, one of which may be an amniocentesis (please see the section on amniocentesis later in this chapter for detailed information about this test).

An increased-risk result does not mean that your baby definitely has this complication, but it means that further testing should be offered to help provide you with more detailed information. You will be given an appointment to discuss this test before it happens and you will be provided with further information to read. Only a small number of women who are in the increased-risk group will actually be pregnant with a baby who has Down's, Edward's or Patau's syndrome.

If your results show that you have an increased risk for Alpha fetoprotein (AFP), an ultrasound is usually done to confirm your baby's age and to look for more than one baby, or to scan for neural tube defects and other atypical conditions which may also be the cause of the elevated screening test result. If the ultrasound shows a single baby at the approximate age determined by the initial due date with no irregularities, an amniocentesis will be offered to look for evidence of genetic anomalies that may have raised your screening test results. If an abnormally high level of AFP is detected in the amniotic fluid, then this indicates a 90 per cent chance that a serious problem is present. An abnormally low AFP reading may indicate that there is a chromosomal problem. If you are identified as being in the lower risk group for spina bifida or Down's, Edward's or Patau's syndrome it does not guarantee that your baby will not have these syndromes; it just means you have a lower risk of this occurring.

The lower the number, the higher the risk

So, for example, a '1 in 180 risk' means there is a higher chance than with a '1 in 400 risk' of your baby having a complication. Please try to keep in mind that even with a 1 in 4 chance (25 per cent) of an affected baby, you still have a higher chance (75 per cent) of having a healthy baby than of having one who has the condition you have been screened for. This is simply a risk result based on a screening test: it is not a definitive result. Definitive positive or negative results can only be obtained through further testing. You will be offered further tests if you receive an 'increased risk' screening result and this testing will be done on your baby while it is inside your body. This is not something you have to have done if you feel that you do not wish to have any other information and are prepared to wait until your baby is born before further testing is done.

Diagnostic testing ('yes' or 'no' answers)

Screening options as described above give healthcare practitioners a baseline to judge if it is appropriate to offer you a diagnostic test, because these tests carry a risk of miscarriage. This risk of miscarriage varies between hospitals but the national average is one miscarriage for every 200 tests done. A diagnostic test can give you a 'yes' or 'no' answer in relation to whether your baby has an irregularity. It cannot promise that your baby is perfect, as it can't detect structural anomalies or all possible congenital conditions, though detailed scans can pick up many major structural issues. Before you decide to have any diagnostic test you must think about how you will feel if you are told your baby has a significant difference and what steps you may wish to take, as a termination of your pregnancy will be offered, even though many chromosomal abnormalities are compatible with life. You will need to consider how you would care for and cope with a disabled baby, child and eventual adult if you chose this option instead of termination, and also look into what schooling and support services are available locally.

Amniocentesis

An amniocentesis is the testing of a small amount of the amniotic fluid surrounding your baby. It provides very reliable information about:

- Blood incompatibilities between mother and baby

- Chromosomal abnormalities

- Certain irregularities related to the growth of the brain and/or the spinal cord, such as spina bifida

- The gender of your baby.

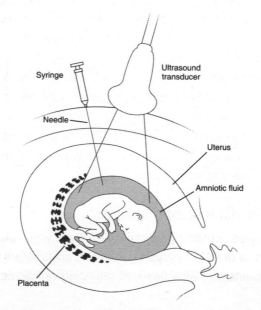

Syringe

Ultrasound transducer

Needle

Uterus

Amniotic fluid

Placenta

Amniocentesis is generally done in combination with ultrasound to prevent injury to your baby and to the umbilical cord and placenta while inserting the needle to remove a sample of the fluid that surrounds your baby. Only a small amount of fluid is taken and your body rapidly replaces it. This fluid contains cells that can be grown in a laboratory, where they are examined to check the number of chromosomes (which carry the genetic code) to see if the number and pattern is standard.

Amniocentesis is considered 99.5 per cent safe, but it does carry an *associated* risk of miscarriage. This means that it isn't known if it directly causes miscarriage, but women have been known to have miscarriages up to a month after an amniocentesis. The national rate for associated miscarriage averages around 1:100, and therefore it is not offered as a routine test.

You need to have a moderately full bladder and to lie still for at least 20 minutes during the amniocentesis. You must try to endure the discomfort of maintaining one position as the test requires quite precise positioning of the needle. The needle itself is only in place for a few seconds before it is withdrawn, leaving behind a thin plastic tube through which the fluid is drawn up. If you have negotiated an agreement with your doctor that you can move at some point during the amniocentesis, then this will be the time when he or she is most likely to encourage you to shift slightly to ease those muscles. Try not to squeeze too hard when offered a comforting hand to hold or you may do some damage to the fingers clutched in yours!

Chorionic villus sampling (CVS)

CVS involves obtaining a sample from your placenta for chromosome or DNA analysis. Chorionic villus refers to the part of the placenta that attaches it to the lining of the uterus, and it is from this area that placental tissue is removed to perform the chromosome test.

CVS is usually offered to women who already know they are at risk of having a baby with a genetic condition. A genetic condition is an inherited one that is carried in the family, such as muscular dystrophy or cystic fibrosis. CVS may also be useful for women who have previously had a baby with a chromosomal disorder such as Down's syndrome, or who are at increased risk because of their age, although most women have amniocentesis to test for these disorders. The only, but significant, advantage of CVS over amniocentesis for chromosomal disorders is that the results are available earlier in the pregnancy. CVS is usually done between 10.5 and 13 weeks of pregnancy, although there are situations where it is performed later.

About 1 in 50 women who have this test will have a miscarriage. About half of these are due to the test itself and the other half would have happened anyway, but it is often impossible to be sure of the cause. There have been a small number of reports in medical journals that CVS may be linked to the risk of limb abnormalities, and that this may be more of a risk if the CVS is done before 9 weeks of pregnancy. However, all CVS tests are followed up by a full, detailed anatomy scan at around 20 weeks of pregnancy to check your baby.

What happens during the trans-abdominal CVS (through your tummy)

If the doctor chooses to use the trans-abdominal approach, your abdomen will be cleaned with antiseptic and a local anaesthetic may be injected into the area where the sampling needle is to go. The sampling needle is then put in and guided into the placenta. This part of the test usually lasts less than a minute, but will undoubtedly feel much longer to the person who is having it done to them.

What happens during the trans-cervical CVS (through the neck of your uterus)

If the doctor chooses to use this method because of the position of your placenta, a speculum will be put into your vagina to help the doctor to see your cervix. This is the same instrument that is used when you have a cervical smear. A very thin type of forceps is passed along the inside of your cervix and into the placenta to take a sample.

In both cases an ultrasound machine is used so that the needle or forceps can be correctly positioned at all times.

Test results

The test results can take anywhere from three to fourteen days to come back, depending upon which technique is being used by the laboratory. The three-day result only reports on Down's, Edward's and Patau's syndromes, so you will still need to wait fourteen days for the complete chromosomal report.

If you have heavy bleeding and/or severe cramping pains after your amniocentesis test (or at any time during your pregnancy), you should contact your maternity hospital immediately.

For more details about any of the screening and diagnostic tests in this book please visit **www.djkirkby.co.uk/my-mini-midwife**, where you will find links to the most up-to-date leaflets available.

COMMON CHANGES DURING PREGNANCY

Pregnancy is a miraculous time of constant change for you and your baby. During the second and third trimesters of your pregnancy you will continue to experience physical and emotional changes. Some symptoms are natural, while others may be warning signs of complications.

Breasts

Right from the beginning your breasts may be larger, firmer and more tender than usual. The areola (the darker area around your nipples) may get larger and grow darker in colour. Halfway through your pregnancy, your breasts may start to leak clear, creamy or yellow fluid (colostrum) in small amounts. Towards the end of your pregnancy, you may want to put gauze or breast pads inside your bra to protect your clothes. The veins right under your skin may become more noticeable too. This is caused by an increased blood supply preparing your breasts for milk production. If you are planning to breastfeed your baby, for most women no special nipple preparation is required. If you have excessively inverted nipples then you may need to do some preparation in order to be ready to breastfeed and your GP or midwife will be able to advise you further if it is agreed that this is required for the position of your nipples. For all pregnant women it is recommended that you wash your breasts and nipples with warm water only – no soap – and dry them well.

Urination

When your uterus expands, it puts pressure on your bladder, meaning you need to urinate more often. Don't try to control this by drinking less fluid: you need to drink at least 1.5 litres of liquids a day. You are more likely to need to urinate more often than normal in early pregnancy while your body is adjusting to the pregnancy hormones, and also as you are nearing the end of your pregnancy (when the baby is pressing on your bladder) the need to find a toilet is likely to be even more frequent, and perhaps even urgent.

Nausea

Some women suffer with 'morning' sickness and some women are never nauseated. 'Morning' sickness isn't necessarily confined to the morning hours. For some women it is an all-day problem during the first 12–14 weeks and for some (very unlucky) women it doesn't pass until after their baby is born. Happily, for most women, the nausea has passed by four months of pregnancy. Try eating smaller meals of simple and mild foods, avoiding spicy and highly acidic foods, and rest in a semi-reclined position immediately after eating, for just a few minutes. If your nausea is more severe than this, try eating a dry cracker (rye is very nourishing) just before getting up in the morning. Sometimes a little bland food in the stomach will help settle your stomach enough that you will be able to hold down your breakfast later. You need to eat well to grow a healthy baby. Take your antenatal vitamins or iron with food during the day when nausea is less of a problem, and always try to take iron with a piece of fruit or small glass of fruit juice as the vitamin C helps you to absorb the iron more efficiently.

'Morning' sickness survival tips

- Flat ginger beer is a traditional remedy. Ginger beer with a stronger 'bite' seems to work better.

- Drinking flat lemonade (or smelling a lemon) may help settle your stomach if ginger beer doesn't work.

- If you are too nauseated to stomach anything, then you can sprinkle a few drops of ginger essential oil on a flannel and inhale the vapours until the nausea eases and then try to drink something.

- Crackers are another option that some women favour as a method of settling their stomach.

- If crackers do not work or get boring, try crisps. They are a good source of potassium but be aware of their high salt and fat content.

Basically you should try to quench your thirst and settle your stomach with healthy and safe foods that you may be craving. So, crisps and soft drinks are acceptable in sensible amounts because you need the fluids and nutrients, but try to balance them out with healthy food and drinks whenever possible.

Try to avoid dehydration. A small glass of ice chips or a tray of watermelon cubes counts for about 250 ml of fluid.

Make a list of odours which trigger nausea and if you work in an open-plan environment, it might be an idea to politely inform colleagues about your nausea triggers and ask for their consideration during the pregnancy. If the smell of certain foods is abhorrent during pregnancy you may want to get help with tasks such as grocery shopping, and if you care for young children you might need help when it comes to changing smelly nappies.

During winter months, if you are chilly put on layers that you can easily peel off instead of turning up the heat. Heat and stale air can aggravate the nausea.

Medication is occasionally prescribed for severe vomiting in pregnancy (which is known as hyperemesis gravidarum), but this is usually reserved for those women who have significant vomiting or dehydration. If the vomiting has been excessive enough to dehydrate them and put their own health and their pregnancy at risk, then anti-sickness injections can be prescribed if all other options have failed.

Excessive salivation

This condition is caused by excessive secretion of the salivary glands in the mouth, and is quite annoying and difficult to treat. It tends to diminish in the latter half of pregnancy. Dry cracker snacks can be helpful with this condition, but keep in mind that you do not want to increase your salt and calorie intake too much.

Heartburn

Heartburn is another common complaint of pregnant women, although it isn't your heart that is burning: it's caused by stomach acid. This is common indigestion, but it can still be an aggravation. It's all right to use antacid preparations, but do not use baking soda (sodium bicarbonate) preparations for your heartburn. Before you buy an over-the-counter remedy, ask your midwife, GP or pharmacist which product is recommended. In severe cases of heartburn, you might want to elevate the head of your bed to encourage your stomach fluids to stay put! (Ask your partner to add 8 cm of books to elevate the head of the bed.) You can reassure your partner that this will not affect their sleep: it looks high but it isn't noticeable once you are lying down.

Constipation

Keeping your fluid intake up is one simple way to avoid constipation during pregnancy. You should also exercise every day to help your body process food more efficiently. Try all the natural remedies for constipation first, including extra water, dried and fresh fruit and lots of vegetables as part of your daily diet. If none of these natural techniques improve the problem, ask your GP to prescribe a very mild laxative or stool softener. Don't be shy about discussing this problem; it is simply a by-product of your pregnancy.

Shortness of breath

This may be a problem once the baby is large enough to interfere with your breathing muscles. It can sometimes be caused by things other than your growing baby, such as low iron levels or more serious conditions, so you may need to seek advice from your midwife or GP if you experience shortness of breath. A first step to alleviate the condition is to try slowing down your movements and practising deep breaths from the chest. If you still have trouble breathing, or if you have any chest or back pain along with the shortness of breath, then this should be considered an emergency – call for an ambulance and ask for a paramedic to attend. Please note that if ambulance services are aware you are pregnant then a paramedic will be sent with the ambulance.

Backache

You may experience backaches due to the added weight gain from your pregnancy, but that isn't the only reason your back may hurt. As your uterus grows, your pelvic bone joints relax, which can cause pain in your lower back. This change in the tension of your pelvic joints is due to the work of the hormone relaxin, which allows your body to adapt to your pregnancy. Comfortable shoes may help, and good posture too, but more than anything else, exercise will probably relieve your backache and prevent it coming back. Strong muscles can take more stress before they become strained. Develop a routine of back exercises every day from the beginning of your pregnancy. Your midwife or GP will be happy to advise you.

Sciatica

Towards the end of the pregnancy some women feel that the baby is pushing on a nerve in their back; this sensation is often called sciatica. This pain can be concentrated in your back or shoot down one or both legs, making walking more difficult. To try and relieve this pressure you can get on your hands and knees, which will encourage your baby's weight to fall towards the floor. You can also try getting on your knees and resting your forearms on the floor, or sitting straddled front-to-back on a chair so your arms support you on the backrest. Use this position when you are watching TV or reading to encourage your baby into the optimum position for late pregnancy and delivery. This will relieve the pressure on your back as your baby shifts, and may give you a lot of backache relief. A warm bath and hot or cold compresses (a hot water bottle, wheat bag or bag of frozen vegetables) sometimes work, too.

Insomnia

Early in your pregnancy you may be very sleepy and feel as if you are sleeping all the time, and then at the end of your pregnancy you will wish those days were back again. Most often trouble with sleeping comes from the difficulty of finding a comfortable sleeping position. For example, if you have always slept on your stomach, you won't be able to do so by the middle of your pregnancy.

However, even the simple act of turning over at night later on in your pregnancy can become a task of monumental proportions, as it may take you several separate motions to do what used to be one fluid movement. This is all because your hips are loosening up in preparation for allowing your baby to pass through during birth and your stomach muscles have relaxed in order to accommodate your baby as it grows.

Later on in your pregnancy shortness of breath, restless legs or heartburn may aggravate insomnia, so prop yourself or your bed head up at night. Shortness of breath that comes on suddenly, that gets worse or that does not ease on resting needs to be investigated by a doctor. Also, an active baby can help keep you awake, and you are much more aware of your baby's movements at night as you have time to concentrate on them. To keep your baby and yourself as calm as possible at night don't drink caffeinated beverages in the evening after supper. Try a soothing herbal tea such as chamomile after your third month of pregnancy has passed. It is best to wait until the first three months of pregnancy have passed before drinking herbal teas that are safe in pregnancy, because there is not enough conclusive research to prove that they are safe for every pregnancy before this time.

Exercising a few hours before you go to bed may help you rest easier, or a warm bath may do the same thing. It is important not to drink alcohol or take sleeping pills to try to solve your insomnia; there are safer solutions. Just ask your midwife or GP for more advice.

Skin changes

Many women get very upset about changes in the colour of their skin, but these changes are common. Your skin may simply look 'flushed', as if you are blushing, or you may develop brownish markings on your face. Some women get a dark line down the middle of their abdomen, where the skin darkens considerably from the navel to the pubic hair. This will fade or disappear entirely after birth. Acne crops up to plague some women; in others acne may actually be improved during pregnancy. Changing hormone levels are responsible for these skin colour changes, but they usually all go away or fade dramatically after your baby is born.

Varicose veins

Varicose veins, or 'varicosities', are caused when the veins in your legs and elsewhere (see the section on haemorrhoids below) get weak and enlarge with blood. They have to work harder to carry blood back up your legs to your heart. Sometimes pregnancy can aggravate this problem, because your uterus partially cuts off circulation from your legs as it increases in size. Exercise will help your veins to work better because as your muscles work while you exercise they will help move fluid back up your legs. I expect by now you have probably noticed that I highly recommend exercise as a solution to many things!

Try not to stand without moving for long periods of time. When you sit, try to prop your legs up to make return circulation easier and paddle your feet back and forth and swirl them round from time to time. Varicose veins can be more of a problem for women having their second or third child. But even if you are having your first baby, try to do as much as you can to help the circulation in your legs.

Support tights can be a big help, but avoid all tight clothing such as knee-high stockings, because they will only cut off circulation more.

Haemorrhoids

Many women suffer with haemorrhoids, or get haemorrhoids for the first time, while they are pregnant, but this doesn't necessarily have to happen to you.

Haemorrhoids are enlarged veins right at the opening of the rectum. Though they are sometimes due to the blockage of circulation caused by the increased size of the baby you are carrying, they can also be caused by the straining due to constipation. Keep your fluid intake up to help avoid constipation.

If you do suffer with haemorrhoids, try lying on your side with your hip elevated on a pillow to help your blood circulate away from this area with ease during the night. Soaking in a warm bath can help, too, and you can use over-the-counter remedies such as witch-hazel wipes which help cool the area, reduce the itching and pain and shrink the haemorrhoids. Before you buy moist wipes be sure to ask if all the ingredients in them are safe for your baby. The medication in ointments is frequently absorbed through the skin and may affect your baby. If you suspect your haemorrhoids are bleeding, call your GP or midwife.

Prevention is the word here! Eat well and add fruits, raw vegetables, bran products and lots of water to your diet every single day. See the section 'Adopt a healthier lifestyle' in 'The Twelve-Month Pregnancy' chapter for more information.

Vaginal discharge

You may notice more vaginal discharge than usual during your pregnancy. This mucus secretion occurs from the cervix in response to the hormones of pregnancy and helps to keep harmful bacteria at safe levels. Mucus secretion is different from leaking of amniotic fluid. All this is quite normal and there really isn't much that can be done to change the situation. If you feel your discharge is excessive, or that it has a bad odour, then it should be checked by your GP.

Many women seem to get thrush infections while they are pregnant that need treatment (have I mentioned how glamorous pregnancy is?!), but they are not harmful to your baby. A simple safe treatment for thrush infections during pregnancy is natural live yogurt. Spread it on the itchy area and enjoy the soothing relief. Use this treatment as often as you need to, in combination with wearing cotton underwear and loose clothing for at least three days; if you are not completely better then, see your GP. If you experience discharge that is watery or comes in gushes, put a maternity pad on and call your local maternity hospital.

Abdominal pain/round ligament pain

Especially during the latter half of pregnancy, when the uterus and your baby are growing larger, you may experience lower abdominal discomfort. One source is round ligament pain. Round ligaments are cord-like structures that originate beneath the groin region and extend to the top of the uterus on both sides.

Round ligament pain is described as a sharp pain in either or both groin regions and is caused by stretching and spasms of the round ligaments. Sudden movements, like rolling over in bed or walking, may aggravate round ligament pain. Reduced physical activity, application of warm heat or the use of a pregnancy support belt may help. Constipation can also cause abdominal pain. If abdominal pain is severe, comes in waves or is continual, please call your local maternity hospital. There can be other more serious causes, which are discussed in the 'Less Common Changes and Complications during Pregnancy' chapter.

Symphysis pubis discomfort

This will affect most women to a mild degree towards the end of their pregnancy and is related to the cartilage between your pubic bone softening and allowing more movement there than you are used to. There is another, more debilitating condition called symphysis pubis dysfunction which affects relatively few women in pregnancy and for which they will require additional care and support. If you are at all concerned, please contact your midwife to discuss it further.

Cravings

It's important to keep eating your balanced diet, no matter what your cravings are. If you feel like eating a whole bag of spinach at 2 a.m., then wash it well and eat it raw or cooked. If you keep craving things (even healthy foods like vegetables), then you may have a nutritional deficiency which needs correcting, so in this case it would be advisable to speak to your midwife or GP. If you feel like eating hot chilli or a packet of biscuits, then that's another issue and one that needs to only be given into in moderation.

Pica

This is the medical term for the unusual cravings for non-food items such as clay, ice or washing powder that you might have while you are pregnant. No one knows quite why this happens, but some women experience it and it can be harmful. Please contact your midwife or GP if you experience this.

Dizzy spells

Some pregnant women do faint. This is caused by the circulation changes happening in your body, and it usually goes away by the second half of pregnancy. Lying on your back towards the end of pregnancy may also cause dizziness because your baby is lying on a large blood vessel that runs along your spine. This is why resting and sleeping on your left side is recommended, because this moves your baby off the blood vessel that runs down your back past your womb; this vessel has an important job to do because it carries oxygen around your body. It is slightly over to the right side of your back, and the weight of your growing baby is more likely to put pressure on it if you lie on your right side. Don't suddenly change positions, such as going from lying to standing, as this can also cause you to faint. When you are lying down, ease yourself up to a standing position in stages. This will give your body time to adjust to the new position.

The reason why you faint is because if your brain suddenly loses a lot of its blood supply, the fastest way it can equalise the supply is by throwing you to the floor so your body is horizontal. This means it's less effort for your heart to pump the blood back up to your brain. All quite simple and perhaps less scary when you understand why, but still dangerous if you faint and hit your head. If you feel faint, try to lie down on your left side until the feeling passes. If you do faint, then once you have come round you will need to contact your midwifery team to let them know what has happened, so that they can ascertain whether you require a check-up. If they do want to see you, then they are likely to suggest you make your way to them, and in this case you will need to make sure you have someone who can accompany you should you feel unwell or faint again while you are making your way there.

Swelling

Not infrequently in late pregnancy swelling can occur in the joints and cause pain that feels like arthritis. This is especially seen with women who develop leg swelling during the day and notice stiff, sore finger joints the following morning after resting overnight. More rarely swelling (particularly in your face) can be linked to a condition called pre-eclampsia, and there is a section later on in this book in the 'Less Common Changes and Complications during Pregnancy' chapter which goes into more detail about this pregnancy-related disorder.

A similar situation occurs in carpal tunnel syndrome, where a nerve that supplies sensation to the hands becomes entrapped in a tunnel of swollen tissue. The nerve in question produces numbness in one or both hands, more frequently at night. Both conditions may be improved by salt restriction during pregnancy and the natural fluid loss that occurs after delivery. A hand splint may also be helpful and your GP or physiotherapist will recommend this if needed.

Again, pressure from the growing uterus and your changing hormones can cause swelling, especially in your legs, feet and hands. Some of this is the blockage of drainage pathways in your upper legs which can be caused by the pressure of your baby and by water retention. Be sure to avoid excessive salt intake, which will only make you retain more water. A combination of gentle exercise, support tights and resting with your legs elevated should help a little. If your feet, ankles or legs are swollen and aren't relieved overnight, then ask your partner to place two or three books at the foot of the bed. If the swelling is new or has come on suddenly, make sure you ask your midwife to check your blood pressure. Notify your midwife, GP or obstetrician if swelling increases dramatically or occurs in your face or around your eyes, as this may be an indication of rising blood pressure. See the section on high blood pressure in the 'Less Common Changes and Complications during Pregnancy' chapter for more information.

Stretch marks

Stretch marks show up usually on breasts, the buttocks and lower abdomen, but they can also occur in other places. Moisturising creams probably won't do much to help because stretch marks are caused by the breakdown of elastic tissue right below the skin's surface. Excessive and rapid weight gain will make matters worse, so keeping your weight gain under control through a combination of healthy food choices, portion control and gentle exercise will do more to avoid stretch marks than anything else. The good news is that stretch marks usually change to a pale white within a year or two after pregnancy, and so become less noticeable.

Nosebleeds

Some women have frequent nosebleeds during pregnancy caused by extra blood supply in the nasal lining. A simple treatment to combat a nosebleed is to apply finger pressure on the side of the bleeding nose. Call your maternity hospital if the bleeding is heavy and you are unable to stop it with nasal pressure. Nasal congestion is also a common complaint, but you should avoid nose drops, unless they have been prescribed by your GP or obstetrician.

Headaches

Mild headaches are one of the most common complaints in the first few months of pregnancy. Most headache remedies are not practical in pregnancy or helpful (and you should seek advice from your midwife, doctor or chemist before taking any), although you can use peppermint oil sticks on your forehead or area where the pain is most concentrated. These headaches are caused by blood-circulation changes and will usually stop after the first half of your pregnancy. If you notice the headaches are associated with sensitivity to light, excessive nausea or vomiting, fever, or blurred or sparkling vision, call your maternity hospital immediately.

Braxton Hicks contractions

The uterine muscle can contract spontaneously anytime from early pregnancy until the onset of real labour. Usually the contractions are irregular and painless (Braxton Hicks contractions), but may produce 'false' labour if they become painful. If the contractions become progressively closer together, last longer and become more painful, notify your midwife or local maternity hospital so they can make certain you are not in premature or early labour.

Emotional changes

Many pregnant women may feel downright joyous one minute then burst into tears the next. These up-and-down mood swings are part of the hormonal changes going on in your body. The impending changes in your life can also be quite overwhelming. When any woman gets pregnant she worries about the health of her baby, about the pain of labour and about the future: how she will adjust to being a mother, how it will affect friendships and relationships (for example, if your friends are mostly childless) and countless different issues all associated with the addition of a baby into her life. Please talk to your midwife or GP if you find yourself becoming increasingly anxious or distressed, as there is help that can be offered.

What to do about mood swings

Most of these anxieties can be eliminated by asking questions or just talking about your worries. Expect these mood shifts, and don't think something is drastically wrong when they occur. No matter how much a woman wants a baby, she still may feel inadequate and under-prepared once she becomes pregnant. The key to working through anxiety and depression is to talk about your feelings. So you should communicate your feelings, even if you think they are too embarrassing.

Try not to worry and concentrate on living your life one day at a time. When you feel anxious, try to do something that relaxes you such as reading, pampering yourself with a warm, relaxing bath or whatever else you like to do that calms you. Reach out to others when you need a comforting word. You will be surprised how many people will tell you they have felt the same at some point in their lives; anxiety and depression are not uncommon. If you still feel anxious or depressed, be sure to talk it over with your midwife or GP before it has a chance to affect your overall health.

Sexual changes

With your mood shifts come other emotional changes, too, including your feelings about sex. Desire for sex may rise or fall significantly during pregnancy. If you lose interest in sex, don't worry. It happens to a lot of women and doesn't usually last long. You may find that your partner's sex drive falls dramatically due to his concerns over possibly hurting the baby or being too intimately close to the baby. Reassure him that normal sexual intercourse during a healthy pregnancy will cause no harm to the baby. Be sure to discuss your feelings and have your partner read this book. Remember, pregnancy is a natural process and a woman's body is designed to cope with it and still function as normal in the majority of cases.

Health fact

You only need an extra 200 calories a day when you are pregnant. This is approximately 500g of melon, 200g of turkey, a small pot of fruit yogurt, an apple with a slice of buttered bread or a handful of dried apricots.

 Be money wise

Baked beans and eggs have a lot of protein in them, but are much cheaper and lower in fat than meat. However, it is important to remember that you should only buy eggs that are guaranteed to be salmonella free (in the UK this is indicated by the red lion stamp), and that the eggs must be cooked until the yolk is solid in order to ensure that they are safe to eat while pregnant.

Exercise shortcuts

Swinging on a swing in the park can be good fun and also a workout for your arms, legs and abdominal muscles. Be careful to swing yourself gently so as not to put too much pressure on your abdominal muscles.

ROUTINE ANTENATAL CARE

During your pregnancy, as long as all goes well, you can be expected to be seen by your midwife or GP at the following stages:

First contact with a healthcare professional

This appointment is likely to be the first time you tell a health professional that you are pregnant and therefore should cover topics such as taking folic acid, which foods are safe to eat and how to prepare them, screening and diagnostic tests available to you (including their risks versus benefits), and lifestyle advice about exercise, stopping smoking, stopping recreational drug use and cutting alcohol back to a minimum or cutting it out completely.

Booking appointment (ideally by 10 weeks)

At your booking appointment the midwife should:

- give you information on pregnancy-specific exercises (such as pelvic floor exercises)

- discuss screening tests again in order to answer any questions you may have and get your consent for the ones you have chosen

- explain to you about the appointments you will be given during a routine pregnancy and identify if you may need extra appointments during your pregnancy (for example, if you have a pre-existing condition such as diabetes)

- discuss the routine blood tests recommended in pregnancy, and then take these with your consent

- measure your height and weight

- discuss the various places you are able to choose to give birth (though these may change during the course of your pregnancy)

- tell you which parenting classes are available

- tell you some issues to look out for during pregnancy, such as depression, and how to spot the early signs

- give you information about maternity benefits.

You should be given information verbally and then also in leaflet form to take away with you. Please ask for leaflets if you are not given any.

16-week check

This is when you can expect the midwife to:

- give you the results of all screening tests done (if any results are outside standard ranges then you will be told before this appointment)

- reassess the planned pattern of care for your pregnancy in case you need additional care

- listen to your baby's heart rate

- measure your blood pressure and test your urine

- discuss the routine anomaly scan, which will be done between 18 and 20 weeks of pregnancy.

18–20-week check

At 18–20 weeks, if you have consented to it, an ultrasound scan should be performed to rule out any structural anomalies on your baby. The position of your placenta will also be checked during this scan to make sure it isn't anywhere near the neck of your womb. If it is, then you will be given another scan at 32 weeks to see how close it is at that time, because it may affect your choice of type of birth.

25-week check

At this appointment you can expect to:

- have your tummy measured from your pubic bone to the fundus (top) of your growing womb, and this measurement will be marked on a chart

- have your blood pressure measured and your urine tested for protein and sugar

- have a chance to chat with your midwife and ask him/her any questions you may have.

28-week check

Here you can expect the midwife to:

- take some more blood tests to make sure everything remains within normal limits

- measure your blood pressure and test your urine for protein and sugar

- measure and plot symphysis (the centre of your pubic bones where they are held together by a section of cartilage) to the top (fundus) of your uterus

- have a chat with you and answer any questions you need to ask.

31-week check

Your midwife will:

- measure your blood pressure and test your urine for protein and sugar

- measure and plot symphysis-to-fundus height

- find out the results of any blood tests done at 28 weeks that were within normal limits (if outside normal range, then you will be told sooner)

- review your plan of care and make sure it is still appropriate for your pregnancy.

34-week check

At 34 weeks, all pregnant women should be seen again, and at this visit you can expect:

- a discussion about what you need to do to prepare for labour and birth, including information that tells you about the various ways in which you can cope with pain in labour and what your birth plan should include

- to find out how to tell if you are in established labour (also see the 'Is This Really Labour?' chapter in this book)

- to be offered a second dose of anti-D if your blood is rhesus-negative (this varies between maternity units, with some only giving one, stronger dose during pregnancy)

- your blood pressure to be measured and your urine tested for protein and sugar

- the midwife to measure and plot symphysis-to-fundus height

- if this is not your first pregnancy, to find out the results of any blood tests done at 28 weeks that were within standard limits (if outside normal range, then you will be told sooner)

- the midwife to review your plan of care and make sure it is still appropriate for your pregnancy.

You may also like to discuss your birth plan with your midwife at this stage.

36-week check

At the 36-week appointment, all pregnant women will be seen again. During this visit you can expect to discuss:

- breastfeeding information, including techniques and good management practices that should help you succeed (find out more in the breastfeeding section in 'The Postnatal Map' chapter of this book)

- how to take care of your new baby

- vitamin K prophylaxis (a medication offered to your baby soon after birth to help with blood clotting) and newborn screening tests

- how to take care of yourself after you have had your baby

- awareness of the difference between 'baby blues' and postnatal depression.

You can also expect the midwife to:

- measure your blood pressure and test your urine for protein and sugar

- measure and plot symphysis-to-fundus height

- check the position of your baby to make sure it is head down

- if your baby is in the breech presentation (bum down), offer you the chance to have an obstetrician try to turn your baby around, which is called external cephalic version (ECV).

38-week check

You can expect:

- your blood pressure to be measured and your urine to be tested

- the midwife to measure and plot your symphysis-to-fundus height

- to get your usual chance to chat to your midwife and ask questions, and he or she should also give you information about your options if you go more than one week over your expected due date.

40-week check

For women having their first pregnancy, an appointment at 40 weeks should be scheduled to:

- measure blood pressure and test urine for protein and sugar

- measure and plot symphysis-to-fundus height.

41 weeks

For women who have not given birth by 41 weeks:

- a membrane sweep will be offered

- an induction of labour appointment will be offered

- blood pressure will be measured and urine tested for protein and sugar

- the midwife will measure and plot symphysis-to-fundus height.

LESS COMMON CHANGES AND COMPLICATIONS DURING PREGNANCY

Pregnancy is a normal state for women, but sometimes complications arise that require immediate attention. Almost all complications give some kind of warning sign and you, or your partner, are likely to be the first to notice a symptom that needs attention. Your blood pressure, urine and weight, the position of your baby and your baby's heartbeat are checked at each appointment with your midwife or GP because changes in these could signal a problem. Problems that are picked up early have the best chance of being treated and cured or controlled.

Call your maternity hospital immediately if you experience any of these symptoms:

- Bleeding from nipples, rectum or bladder, or coughing up of blood

- Vaginal bleeding, no matter how small the amount

- Swelling of hands or face

- Dimness or blurring of vision

- Severe or continuous headaches

- Abdominal pains that don't go away or that become more frequent or painful

- Chills, or fever over 40 degrees

- Persistent vomiting

- Painful or burning urination

- Decreased fetal movements

- Sudden or steady loss of fluid from the vagina.

Early-pregnancy bleeding

There are many causes of bleeding during pregnancy and these vary depending upon when the bleeding occurs. If you experience bleeding early in your pregnancy, you will be sent for a scan to determine the cause. Two serious causes of early-pregnancy bleeding are miscarriage and ectopic pregnancy. Two minor causes of early-pregnancy bleeding are post coital (after lovemaking) and cervical erosion.

Miscarriage

This is the most common serious cause of early bleeding. Most miscarriages cannot be prevented; they are nature's way of dealing with pregnancies that are not developing properly. A miscarriage is usually characterised by bleeding more than you would normally experience during a heavy period and is usually associated with cramping, but you may sometimes feel the cramping without noticing any bleeding. An ectopic pregnancy, or the implantation of a fertilised egg outside the uterus (usually in a fallopian tube), is another serious cause of early bleeding.

Ectopic pregnancies

These are almost always associated with pain in one side of your upper groin area (see the chapter on 'Conception and Moving Forward' for other symptoms). Most of the bleeding is internal, which can be life-threatening because of its hidden nature. Call your local maternity hospital immediately if you experience severe abdominal pain early in your pregnancy, abdominal pain combined with pain in your shoulders or any abdominal pain that comes and goes in 'waves' or is associated with bleeding.

Late-pregnancy bleeding

Bleeding late in pregnancy can be serious, but the most common cause is a 'bloody show', one of the first signs of labour. This is caused by the thinning of the cervix and is usually combined with thick mucus. Cervical irritation, for example through sexual intercourse, as well as pre-existing cervical erosion and pelvic exams, which can irritate the cervix (which has increased blood supply during pregnancy), can also cause bleeding.

The most serious late-pregnancy bleeding is caused by either placenta praevia or placental abruption. When these conditions occur, they happen most often in the final three months of the pregnancy. Placenta praevia results when your placenta partially or completely covers your cervix. As your cervix thins in preparation for labour, it will stretch any placental tissue attached to it and bleeding will occur. The other serious cause of late bleeding, placental abruption, occurs when the placenta separates from the inner lining of your uterus before your baby is born. This is usually accompanied by sudden, severe abdominal pain. Either condition can lead to the death of your baby and serious harm to you. Do not ignore any pain that is sudden and/or severe in onset.

You must be sensible and avoid the urge to try to be stoic if experiencing pain during pregnancy. Let the professionals decide if there is a problem if you are not sure; that is what we are paid for.

If you experience significant bleeding in your pregnancy, you may be hospitalised for observation and evaluation. If the bleeding is serious or if the fetal monitor shows a persistent, non-reassuring fetal heart-rate pattern, a caesarean delivery may be required.

Please be reassured by the fact that most bleeding is the result of minor causes that require no treatment. It is important, however, for you to know that bleeding can indicate serious problems. You should report all bleeding to your local maternity hospital or GP immediately, so that the severity of this blood loss and the well-being of both you and your baby can be assessed.

High blood pressure in pregnancy

Pregnant women can develop pre-eclampsia, which is a syndrome associated with high blood pressure known as pregnancy-induced hypertension (PIH). The exact cause of these potentially serious conditions is unknown, but they are thought to be linked to how your placental arteries form early in your pregnancy.

When changes of blood pressure are detected early, you and your baby can avoid serious problems. However, with PIH you will often feel quite well, except for possible headaches in the beginning. This is one of the reasons why attending regular, scheduled antenatal appointments is so important. Pre-eclampsia can cause damage to multiple organs in your body if undetected. Your baby can suffer from a lack of oxygen and nutrients, which can lead to growth problems, ongoing health problems throughout life or even death.

Women who are overweight, diabetic or over 40 years old are considered to be at an increased risk of developing this complication of pregnancy. Mothers with kidney disease, twins or a history of high blood pressure are also considered to be likely candidates.

High blood pressure is caused when the blood vessels in the body contract. This increases the pressure and lessens the amount of blood flowing to the uterus and placenta and to your baby. Mild changes in blood pressure for a brief period are unlikely to cause problems. However, prolonged and severe spasms of the vessels can be potentially harmful and need closer monitoring (and sometimes drug treatment for some women) in order to lower the blood pressure.

A sudden weight gain or noticeable swelling of the face and hands can indirectly signal high blood pressure. If this is the case with you, then mention it to your midwife, GP or obstetrician so they are aware of this fact. What you are looking for is swelling that isn't normal for you and is particularly noticeable, such as swelling in your face.

Some women experience no distinct symptoms at all. Headaches, visual disturbances or pain in the upper abdomen or back may indicate a more serious problem and you should call your local maternity unit if any of these occur. By monitoring your blood pressure, weight and urine at each antenatal visit, your midwife, GP or obstetrician should be able, in most cases, to make an early diagnosis of the problem and take steps to help you avoid serious complications.

Each case of PIH and pre-eclampsia is treated differently, depending upon a variety of factors. However, the eventual birth of your baby will speed your recovery from this disorder. If you have needed medicating during your pregnancy to help stabilise your blood pressure, then you may need to continue taking these tablets for a period of time during your postnatal period. Most of the medication used in pregnancy is safe to continue to use when breastfeeding, but do not be afraid to ask this question for clarity.

Fluid retention

Certain foods and liquids contain an excessive amount of salt, which promotes increased fluid retention in some women. You may want to consider cutting the following out of your regular diet:

* bacon, sausage, ham, pork and lunchmeats

* salted butter and condiments such as soy sauce, oyster sauce, mustard, ketchup and brown sauce

* tinned soups, vegetables, meat and fish

* salted popcorn, pretzels, potato crisps, nachos, salted nuts, etc.

* tomato juice, bouillon/stock cubes, additional salt with meals.

Premature labour

Labour usually occurs some time after the 37th week of pregnancy (37–42 weeks is considered full term). A baby born before 37 weeks is considered premature. These infants may require special care in breathing and maintaining their body temperatures, or they may be perfectly able to do these without help. Each baby will be assessed as an individual at birth, whether born prematurely or not.

Warning signs of premature labour

Signs and symptoms include:

- Uterine contractions – more than four in one hour

- Period-type cramps – these may come and go, or be constant

- Abdominal cramps – with or without diarrhoea

- Low backache – which comes and goes, or remains constant

- Pelvic pressure – feeling like your baby is pushing down

- Change in vaginal discharge – a sudden increase in amount, or if it becomes more mucus-like, watery, slightly bloody, neon yellow or green tinged.

If you have one or more of these symptoms, you might be in premature labour. You should call your local maternity hospital immediately for advice. They will likely invite you in to check you and your baby over and observe you for a while before making a decision about what care to offer you.

Atypical antibodies and prevention of haemolytic disease in the newborn

Are you sitting comfortably, dear reader? There is no way to make this topic interesting, so you may as well settle yourself down somewhere with lots of cushions, just in case you fall asleep while reading this boring, but vitally important, information.

You will be offered a series of routine blood tests at one of your first antenatal visits. One of these will be to determine your blood type and Rh factor. The most common blood type is type O; the most common Rh factor is positive. People with type O, B, A, or AB positive blood have a positive Rh factor. Those with type O, B, A, or AB negative blood have a negative Rh factor. Still awake? OK, then read on...

When your blood type is Rh negative, and your baby's father's is Rh positive, your baby may inherit the father's positive blood type, which could cause a problem during pregnancy. If your blood type is Rh negative, your body's immune system will recognise the baby's Rh positive blood cells that escape into your circulation. As you now know, these cells are different from yours. Because they are different from yours, your body will produce antibodies to destroy your baby's red blood cells.

These newly formed antibodies may not be a problem during your first pregnancy; however, they can lead to a serious disease in any subsequent pregnancies. This is known as haemolytic disease of the newborn (HDN). For these reasons, the blood test I mentioned at the beginning of this section checks for antibodies, and if any are found, they are monitored closely throughout your pregnancy.

HDN can be prevented in most cases by giving you an injection of anti-D, which prevents your immune system from reacting to your baby's red blood cells. The anti-D finds your baby's red cells in your circulation and throws a chemical cloak over them so you don't produce antibodies against them.

If your blood type is found to be Rh negative, the option of anti-D should be discussed with you. Your consent is needed to give you this injection and you need to be aware that it is a blood product, albeit a very small amount of technically 'safe' blood. However, some religious beliefs discourage the administration of blood products, no matter how small, and there can never be a guarantee that the blood is perfectly safe, as diseases which are unknown at this time or that we are unable to look for may be present in the anti-D. This injection is routinely offered to women with Rh negative blood during pregnancy and within 72 hours following birth.

Group B streptococcus (GBS)

GBS is a common bacteria which can be found in many women, most commonly in the vagina or rectum, which can sometimes cause serious medical problems for your baby. It is not routinely screened for during pregnancy because it can appear and disappear throughout your pregnancy, and therefore there is no set time when it can be accurately screened for.

If GBS is detected during pregnancy, usually when a swab is taken if you've 'broken' your waters, then treatment can be offered. Long-term protection cannot be guaranteed because you can become positive again for GBS after treatment and before your baby is born. The best way to prevent GBS infection is the use of intravenous antibiotics during labour. If you are found to have GBS in pregnancy, are known to have had this infection in previous pregnancies, or have any of the risk factors below, then your options for treatment will be discussed with you.

Mothers at increased risk for GBS are those:

- with fever during labour

- with a previous baby/child with a GBS infection

- with prolonged ruptured membranes ('broken waters').
  The definition of 'prolonged' varies between expert groups such as NICE and the Royal College of Obstetricians and

Gynaecologists (RCOG), with the earliest classification of 'prolonged' being 18 hours after your membranes have ruptured. Your hospital should tell you what their definition of prolonged is, and their policy on what to do when you phone to tell them that your waters have broken, but please ask if you are not told.

- with rupture of membranes before reaching 37 weeks of pregnancy

- going into labour before 37 weeks of pregnancy.

Please visit **www.djkirkby.co.uk/my-mini-midwife**, where you will find links to the most up-to-date information about GBS available. If you have further questions about this condition, then your midwife, GP or health visitor will be happy to answer them for you.

Health fact

Iron can be found in large amounts in dried fruit, red meat, broccoli and dried beans. Iron is important because it helps your blood carry oxygen around your body, and the more oxygen you are able to carry, the more you will be able to share with your baby. Vitamin C aids in iron absorption, so you should include fruit or juice when eating foods which contain iron. Remember that iron is easily destroyed by cooking so eat raw (salads) or lightly steamed leafy green vegetables (such as spinach and kale) every day. Avoid taking iron with drinks containing milk, because milk will reduce the amount of iron your body can absorb.

Be money wise

Investigate what maternity benefits are available to you. If you go to www.gov.uk/browse/working/time-off you will find links to information to help you work out your maternity pay, benefits, maternity/paternity leave and other useful information. Once you find out how much money you will have coming in, then you can budget accordingly and have time to get used to having a lower income.

Gestational diabetes and the glucose tolerance test

There are several kinds of diabetes, all relating to the delicate balance of sugar (glucose) in the blood. Insulin is a hormone that converts glucose into the body's main source of energy, called glycogen. When the body fails to use insulin in the right way or doesn't produce enough of it, then the level of sugar in the blood becomes too high, which can be dangerous for you and your baby. In pregnancy some women may develop diabetes just for the duration of the pregnancy. This is called gestational diabetes and means your blood sugar has risen and is staying above acceptable levels during your pregnancy.

Some women are more likely to develop gestational diabetes than others, particularly those who have previously delivered a large baby (one weighing more than 4.5 kg), and women who are obese. Gestational diabetes can cause the baby to grow bigger during pregnancy than normal, which may lead to a difficult vaginal birth or a caesarean delivery. Babies born to gestational diabetics are also prone to having low blood sugar levels and jaundice for a few days or more after delivery. Women who have had stillborn babies or who have a family history of diabetes are also thought to be more likely to develop gestational diabetes.

Pregnant mothers with gestational diabetes may develop a condition where there is too much fluid surrounding the baby (polyhydramnios), which can cause premature labour and increase the risk of respiratory distress syndrome in the baby. Women with gestational diabetes are also more susceptible to urinary tract infections and high blood pressure.

At every antenatal check all women will have their urine checked for glucose, and if you have this or any risk factors for gestational diabetes, you may be offered a blood test to monitor your fasting glucose levels at around 28 weeks of pregnancy. If this shows that you have a higher than expected glucose level you will be offered a glucose tolerance test.

Glucose tolerance test (GTT)

Try not to worry if your midwife or doctor recommends that you have a GTT, because most results are within normal limits. For the GTT, a blood test will be taken on your arrival to check your fasting blood sugar level, which means you will need to fast for the 12 hours before the blood test (this is safe to do in this instance). Then you will be given a sugary drink followed by a second blood test two hours after you have drunk this. This test will check how your body has coped with the sugar in the drink. Based on these results, a decision will be made about your body's ability to process sugar and a plan for your care during your pregnancy will be discussed with you.

Most gestational diabetics can control their sugar levels with gentle exercise and a modified diet. However, for some women the solution is not so simple, and they may require monitoring throughout their pregnancy to try to stop the baby from becoming too big. Occasionally, insulin injections are required to control sugar levels, but unlike many other medications, they are completely safe for your baby, as insulin does not cross the placenta.

A modified diet during pregnancy is a sensible option even without diabetes. As discussed earlier, you should try to eat smaller and more frequent meals, including a source of protein and plenty of non-starchy vegetables. Eat wholegrain versions of rice, pasta, bread and cereal. Make your plate look like a rainbow with a wide variety of coloured foods. Examples include red, yellow and green peppers, red tomatoes, green vegetables, brown and yellow carbohydrates, dark and light meat, fish and so on.

Type 1 and type 2 diabetes

Women with type 1 and type 2 diabetes have high-risk pregnancies in comparison with those without. Pre-conception care and good blood glucose control before and during pregnancy can lower these risks, as well as regular antenatal visits to your diabetic specialist midwife and obstetrician.

The risks are:

- your baby is more likely to be stillborn

- your baby is more likely to die in the first month of life

- your baby is twice as likely to have a major abnormality

- your baby is more likely to be born prematurely

- your baby is twice as likely to weigh over 4 kg at birth and ten times as likely to have Erbs palsy (a type of paralysis experienced by large babies during delivery)

- the majority of women with type 1 and type 2 diabetes have their babies delivered by caesarean section.

Good blood glucose control before and during pregnancy offers you the best chance of decreasing these risks. It is extremely important to avoid an unplanned pregnancy (which would mean you would miss out on the benefits of pre-conception care). You should contact your diabetes care team for pre-conception advice. They will review your current insulin regime and make the necessary adjustments. They will ask you to monitor your blood glucose at least four times a day. Folic acid (5 mg per day) will be prescribed and you should start taking this as soon as you plan a pregnancy and continue until the 12th week of pregnancy.

> ### ⏱️ Exercise shortcuts
>
> *Walking is a great and inexpensive form of exercise, and one that you can do with your partner or best friend. If you walk briskly you will greatly increase the health benefits. Remember to wear low-heeled comfortable shoes, preferably trainers. You don't need to be a dog owner to take advantage of the exercise benefits that come from dog walking. Many dog rescue centres are looking for volunteers to help with walking the dogs in their kennels, but be sure to bring along something to scoop up any dog mess so that your hands do not come into contact with the faeces. Some cities and villages also offer 'health walks' schemes that you can join for free, so search for them on the Internet and find out if there is something like this available to you.*

CHANGES IN THE LAST FEW WEEKS OF PREGNANCY

You can expect more changes in the last weeks of your pregnancy. You will probably feel tired and as if you have been pregnant forever. You are likely to feel heavy, clumsy and out of patience with pregnancy. This is all part of getting ready, and being willing to go through the labour and birth process. The more fed up you get, the more you will convince yourself that you are willing to go through *anything* to get this baby out of you and into the real world. That is your first real step towards preparing yourself for labour and birth.

Engagement

You may notice that your bump is lower than usual. This is when your baby's head or bottom 'drops' or engages into the bony part of your pelvis. When this happens you might be able to breathe more easily, as the pressure on your diaphragm will lessen. However, the waddling gait you may already have developed will now become more pronounced as you instinctively try to widen your hips to make room for your baby's head. You may hear your hips 'creak' as you lie awake in the night. It is not unusual to have your sleep patterns further disturbed by the movements of your baby at this stage and the fact that it now may take you about six separate and distinct movements to turn over in bed. Your midwife will be checking to see if your baby's head has engaged in the opening to your pelvis. This is one way to tell if you will be able to give birth vaginally. You may find this part of the examination particularly uncomfortable, especially if the midwife uses something called a 'Pawlick's grip', where she places a finger and thumb on either side of the lowest part of your baby. Many midwives now only use a two-handed form of this check, which you may find more comfortable. If you feel this or any part of the examination is too uncomfortable, please tell your midwife. By keeping her informed of what you can and cannot cope with you will be helping your midwife to give you the best possible care.

Breast enlargement

Your breasts enlarge even more near the end of the pregnancy, and colostrum may start to seep from them. You can make use of breast pads if you wish and it's important to make sure your bra is comfortable and fits well. You will need to be measured again for your feeding bras. If they do not fit properly, then you will spend more time than you need to pushing yourself back into the cups after you turn over at night. A good-fitting and supportive bra is essential to help prevent discomfort in your upper back, as your shoulders get accustomed to this additional weight.

'Red-hot pokers'

You may experience new types of discomfort during the latter stages of pregnancy which are completely normal. Pressure is sometimes reported in the vaginal area, any time from 32 weeks pregnant right through until delivery. You may also experience shooting pains or a 'red-hot poker' sensation in this area as your baby puts pressure on nerves that run along this area of your body.

Frequent urination

You are likely to feel the need to urinate frequently, and will begin to feel as if you have mapped out your local shops by toilet locations.

(⏱) **Exercise shortcuts**

Try swimming as a form of exercise any time, but you may find it of extra benefit during the second half of pregnancy as a way to take the pressure off your feet and legs.

(💡) **Did you know?**

For healthy, straightforward pregnancies there are a variety of places you can choose to give birth, depending on what is available in your local area, such as your own home, the local maternity unit, a peripheral birth centre or an independent birthing unit.

IS THIS REALLY LABOUR?

Plan to monitor your early labour contractions in the comfort of your own home, because you are likely to cope with your contractions better in your own familiar space. You should prepare to call your midwife when your membranes rupture; this can happen a day or more before the birth of your baby but your midwife still needs to know when this happens so he or she can give you an induction date in case your labour doesn't begin. You should also call your midwife when your contractions are coming regularly, i.e. less than ten minutes apart. It is advisable to call earlier if you are quite a distance from where you intend to give birth.

Very early labour is sometimes called 'false' labour as it can take a few days to become established into regular contractions. It is important to know the difference between established and very early labour. Very early labour involves cramps or contractions of the lower abdomen, similar to established labour, but there are some key differences: very early labour does not cause a change in your cervix, and the pain doesn't come in regular intervals and may disappear altogether if you change positions or walk around.

Some labour contractions cause back pain and some cause lower abdominal pain, or both. Expect to cope quite well with these early contractions; in fact you may not recognise labour pains for what they are to begin with, especially if you feel them in your back but are used to pregnancy-associated back pain. Try to move around, and have a warm bath. Gentle massage may be a comfort to some women or try placing a full, covered hot water bottle against the spot where you feel the contractions the most. Remove the hot water bottle between contractions so that your skin does not get too hot. When you think you are in labour, sit down and time your contractions from the start of one contraction to another for several contractions. There are apps available for many types of mobiles, as well as websites which enable you to easily monitor the frequency and duration of your contractions. Your partner may wish to take on this task, as well as providing support to you in other ways such as gentle massage or simply being nearby to provide comfort if needed. If you find your contractions are evenly spaced, are coming closer and closer together and don't go away if you change position or walk around, then you are probably going into established ('real') labour.

Very early labour (sometimes called 'false' labour)

- No 'bloody show'

- Usually associated with cramp-like pains

- Pains are irregular in strength and not getting closer together

- Walking or changing activity or positions may relieve or stop the pains

- No change in the cervix

- No dilation.

Established ('real') labour

- A 'bloody show' may be the first sign

- Contractions get stronger, occur more frequently and last longer

- Walking or changing activity or position doesn't affect the intensity, duration or frequency of contractions

- Contractions are regular and happen at least every ten minutes, or more often

- Duration of contractions is 30 seconds or more

- Your cervix dilates (opens).

Two things you will be asked about when you phone to say you are in labour:

1. How frequent are your contractions – this is the time from the start of one contraction to the beginning of another.

2. How long are your contractions lasting – this is the time from the start of one contraction to the end of the same contraction.

The first stage of labour is the time from the start of regular contractions to the point at which your cervix is fully dilated. Contractions start off by working to shorten your cervix before it starts to dilate, which is known as effacement. Full effacement is when your cervix has completely shortened. With a first labour, once this has happened your cervix will begin to dilate, but with a second labour the effacement and dilation stages may happen simultaneously. The second stage of labour begins when your cervix is fully dilated at 10 cm. This is when your cervix is open enough for your baby to pass through it without causing any damage. You are likely to feel a lot of pressure and urges to push at this stage, which last until your baby has been born. The third stage of your labour will last from the point that your baby is born until you have delivered your placenta.

Be money wise

If money is a worry, try shopping early in the morning or close to closing time. This is when you are most likely to find the reduced price items which are often still in date for a day or two. Homemade bread is much less expensive than store-bought varieties and very simple to make from ready-to-mix packs.

Exercise shortcuts

Try aqua aerobics instead of land-based exercise classes because the resistance of the water makes your body work harder in a shorter period of time. Take an antenatal class or tell your instructor that you are pregnant so that they can help you to avoid overdoing it.

Did you know?

Pregnancy can cause changes in your shoe size, because pregnancy hormones are specially designed to allow your tissues to stretch. You will need some comfortable low-heeled shoes to start your pregnancy with and you may well need to buy a larger or wider pair as your pregnancy progresses, but your feet will probably return to their pre-pregnancy size afterwards.

PAIN RELIEF

OK, now this is a tricky section to write. The thing is, we are all so different and therefore so are our reactions to the pain of labour and how we interpret and cope with it. Some women need minimal pain relief or no pain relief at all and some want everything going; both of these are absolutely fine. Midwives will be guided by your needs and will tell you what all your options are at the time, as these will vary according to what stage of labour you are in, what position you and your baby are in and what medications you are currently using.

The first part of this chapter focuses on natural pain-relief methods

Breathing

OK, OK, I know we all have to breathe. I am talking about structured, controlled breathing in this instance. Let me explain…

As your contraction begins to build you can inhale slowly and deeply through your nose. Concentrate on how your breath feels as it passes over your throat area. Then gently plug your ears with your index fingers and close your eyes. Exhale slowly, producing a long and continuous humming sound; repeat as often as required. This will distract you from the pain, but also has the added benefit of getting a good flow of oxygen to your hard-working muscles. If you are finding it difficult to concentrate you may wish to ask your partner to help you focus on your breathing.

Relaxation

I have also seen women successfully use the following relaxation techniques:

- Visualisation (you are ambling along a sandy beach, in a meadow, etc.)

- Affirmation (your body is strong, is working well for you, knows what it is doing, etc.)

- Conscious relaxation of tense muscles, non-focused awareness (notice what you see, hear, feel, smell and then forget about it, move on to the next sensation)

- Vocalising (moaning, making single sounds like 'oh, oh', groaning), or prayer.

Mobility

Moving around during labour is often a great help to women. For most women, changing position and the ability to wander around to some extent during labour is almost vital if you want to avoid the discomfort that comes from muscles getting stiff from staying in one position too long. Moving around, even if only to change your position from sitting to standing or to kneeling on all fours, can help to ease your baby deeper into your pelvic outlet, the start of your birth canal. Walking up and down stairs or stepping on and off a step in a sideways movement is thought to also help shift your baby deeper into your pelvic outlet. Some women find that kneeling on all fours or sitting on a birthing stool can help them push more effectively. A bean bag or large ball such as one used for abdominal exercising can be very comfortable to sit on while in labour and will encourage you to sit in a good position too.

TENS

Transcutaneous electronic nerve stimulation (TENS) for labour pain is a hand-held, battery-powered device that sends electrical impulses through your lower back through four electrodes. You control the intensity of the stimulus and are able to boost it during a contraction. The theory behind this is that it blocks some of the pain signals from passing through the 'pain gate' in your spine, thus restricting the amount of pain your brain has to process. In my opinion you will either love or hate this method: if it works for you it will work very well and vice versa. Unlike most of the other pain-relief methods, this device cannot be used in conjunction with hydrotherapy (see below) and you will need to rent one before going into labour, as most hospitals do not have a large enough supply. TENS should not be used before 37 weeks of pregnancy because it can cause alterations in your baby's heart rhythm before this time. The majority of women I have cared for found use of a TENS machine very helpful in letting them feel in control of their labour pain.

Hydrotherapy

The labour/birthing pools used in maternity care are much deeper than a normal household bath, about the depth of a hot tub. There are places where you can hire soft-sided birthing pools for use at home, and many maternity units have at least one birthing pool in their labour ward or midwifery-led unit. However, these birthing pools are in great demand so there is no guarantee that they will be available if you choose to give birth in hospital or in a midwifery-led unit. There are some conditions for which use of the birthing pool is unsuitable and your midwife will be able to tell you if you fall into these criteria. Additionally, you cannot use the birthing pool if you have been given pethidine as a form of pain relief, so you may wish to try the birthing pool before deciding to use pethidine.

The hydrotherapy method of pain relief is immediately reversible. If you do not like it, you can get out and try something else. You can also use alternative pain-relief methods in conjunction with this, such as gas and air, breathing, relaxation and massage. The added buoyancy of the water makes it much easier for you to change positions as well.

Hypnosis

Hypnosis is just a fancy term for being really relaxed, and for really focusing in on just one thing while everything else fades into the background. Hypnosis for birth is proving increasingly popular, and research shows that it can make a difference to birth outcome and your feelings of satisfaction in relation to your birthing experience. Hypnosis is all about the mind's ability to affect the body's reactions. Self-hypnosis is said to be a state of deep relaxation, where the mum remains fully alert and in control throughout. To find out more about hypnobirthing classes near you, go to www.hypnobirthing.co.uk. For more information and birth stories, go to the US website at www.hypnobirthing.com.

Massage

Massage is a good technique to use during labour. It can be especially helpful for women who are unable to change positions easily – say, for example, if they have opted to have an epidural. It is advisable for you and your partner to experiment with massage during your pregnancy to find what pressure you can tolerate and which parts of your body you prefer to have massaged. Some women will find even gentle massage too uncomfortable, and labour is not the right time to discover this. If you are one of them, don't despair. Here are some similar techniques which may work in much the same way as massage for you: hot compresses such as a flannel or hot water bottle placed on your back or wherever else you hurt, or ice packs used in the same way; a warm blanket over your entire body; or a lengthy warm shower (take the shower head off the wall and direct the spray to precisely the area you need it most).

There are other techniques people use for pain relief, including singing. I remember one couple who sang hymns together during each contraction. The only other form of pain relief used by that particular woman was a bit of gas and air for the few contractions that she had just before she pushed her baby's head out.

The following section looks at the methods of pain relief that use drugs to help with the pain of labour and birth

Entonox (gas and air)

This used to be known as 'laughing gas'. It is a combination of oxygen and nitrous oxide and you inhale it through a mouthpiece or face mask. It doesn't really relieve the pain you feel, but it does change how you interpret the pain. It also gives you something to focus on, as you need to breathe it in a certain way and begin to use it at a certain point during your contraction. Your midwife will show you how to use it if you choose to use this method. It can make you feel quite giddy (and a few women feel queasy), but the effects wear off quickly when you stop inhaling it. It is quickly reversible and you can use it in conjunction with hydrotherapy, TENS or pethidine, and in several different positions.

Pethidine

This drug has similar properties to morphine, but is safer to use during labour. It is given by injection and it often affects the vomit centres in your brain, so is usually given with an anti-sickness drug. It should start working within 20 minutes after being injected, and while it won't take your pain away, it does help you feel differently about it. The effects will last a couple of hours.

Pethidine is not available for home births and it does not work well for everyone. Some women really do not like the effects, or say it feels like it put the pain 'on top of them'. Once it is in your body you can only wait for it to wear off, so it is best to ask for a smaller dose when trying it for the first time. It can affect your baby if given too close to the time of birth, so your midwife will want to perform an internal examination to see how dilated you are before injecting pethidine into you.

A few hospitals are trialling the use of diamorphine, so if you labour at one of these maternity units then you may be offered this instead of pethidine as an option for pain relief.

Epidural

This is an injection of local anaesthetic into your lower back. It is the only thing that can 'take away' your pain in labour. All the other types discussed are pain 'relievers'. The anaesthetist punctures a hole in your back with a needle, threads a thin plastic tube in and the needle is removed, leaving a long plastic tube in for the duration of your labour. This is taped to your back to keep it safe and out of the way. It will take about 10–20 minutes for the effects of the epidural to work. This type of pain killer can only be given by a qualified anaesthetist. Epidurals can have some side effects immediately or soon after starting, such as low blood pressure, nausea, dizziness or itching skin.

An epidural will make you feel very numb in your legs and you will not be as mobile as you may wish. However, a few hospitals offer mobile epidurals, where you are able to move around with greater ease and in some cases even walk around.

You may find it difficult to pass urine with an epidural. If this happens to you then a midwife can insert a catheter to release the urine from your bladder. Very occasionally epidurals will have 'windows', where the pain still breaks through, which means that you will feel the contraction in a small area. Epidurals can increase your chances of you needing help to birth your baby, usually in the form of a ventouse or forceps delivery, as you are not able to push as well when you can't feel any sensation.

Epidurals can very occasionally cause bad or severe headaches in the following 24–48 hours after birth, which may be an important deciding factor for those of you who already suffer with headaches. Some people complain of back pain for varying lengths of time after having had an epidural.

Health fact

If you are eating low-fat foods, be sure to check that the sugar levels are reasonable, because sometimes the amount of added sugar will go up in relation to the amount of fat being reduced in order to maintain flavour.

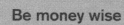 **Be money wise**

Instead of buying lots of pregnancy and baby books, borrow them from friends and family or from your local library.

DIFFERENT WAYS YOU MAY GIVE BIRTH

Every birth is unique. There are a multitude of factors that may influence each form of delivery. Whether your labour has begun naturally or has had to be induced and what kind of monitoring you and your baby need during labour and delivery can also affect how you give birth. To begin with, here is a reminder of the differences between early labour (little or no dilating of the cervix occurs during this phase) and established labour (the time when you should call your midwife if all else is well with you and the pregnancy).

Very early labour (sometimes called 'false' labour)

- No 'bloody show'

- Usually associated with cramp-like pains

- Pains are irregular and not getting closer together

- Walking or changing activity or positions may relieve or stop the pains

- No change in the cervix

- No dilation.

Established ('real') labour

- A 'bloody show' may be the first sign

- Contractions get stronger, occur more frequently and last longer

- Walking or changing activity or position doesn't affect intensity, duration or frequency of contractions

- Cervix dilates

- Contractions are regular and happen at least every ten minutes or more often

- Duration of contractions is 30 seconds or more.

Induction of labour

If you go more than a week over your due date you will be offered a weekly membrane sweep to try and get you to go into labour naturally. This involves having an internal examination, with one finger being used to sweep the membranes around the neck of your womb (cervix). Although this only takes a few minutes to do it feels like a cervical smear, but with more pressure, and some women find it very uncomfortable. You may need to take pain relief after your appointment and/or use a hot water bottle to ease any cramps you may have. Additionally, even though it will likely be the last thing on your mind, you should try the natural induction method at home before a membrane sweep or chemical induction of labour becomes necessary. This involves sexual intercourse in either the 'spoons' or kneeling position, as this allows your body to make use of the natural version of the chemicals in sperm which are chemically replicated for use in the form of pessaries in medical induction. Medical induction of labour may be recommended if you go more than 10–12 days overdue, have prolonged rupture of membranes or have a condition which means it is safer to induce your labour instead of waiting for it to happen naturally.

The best way for you to be induced is to have your waters broken, which is done by the midwife performing a vaginal examination of your cervix. If you are dilated enough she will carefully use a long instrument which looks similar to a crochet hook to tear a small hole in your membranes (this tear will not cause you any pain and the midwife will also protect your baby's head). If this is not enough to put you into established labour then a cannula will be inserted into a vein in your hand or side of your wrist through which a drip containing a drug used to stimulate contractions will be administered.

If labour is induced, the process is increased gradually but may still be more rapid than if your body would have laboured naturally and, as such, your body is not able to build up your endorphin levels to help cope with the pain. Ways you can lessen your pain include walking around the labour room and/or changing your position frequently. Your partner can help by following you with your drip stand, or if you are having your baby's heart beat monitored then he or she may be allowed to manoeuvre the baby monitoring machine around so that you can move about as much as possible. Each contraction will bring you one step closer to getting to hold your baby in your arms, and this thought may help as you progress through your labour.

Monitoring in labour

If your labour has been induced by medical methods it will be recommended that your baby be monitored continuously, as changes in the heart rate pattern may be the first sign of a problem. The belt that holds the monitor against your belly can be uncomfortable or annoying for women and you may need to ask the midwife for 20-minute breaks from the monitor. If your baby is coping well, the midwife can listen in with a hand-held monitor. If you are induced, or need a drip to help your labour progress, the midwife will want to perform vaginal examinations every two hours, instead of the more usual four hours, to make sure the induction or acceleration of the labour is working.

Vaginal birth

The first stage of labour starts with the beginning of your regular contractions and is completed when your cervix reaches 10 cm dilatation. The first stage of labour can take quite a long time, especially with a first baby. It isn't at all uncommon for the first stage of labour to last 12 or more hours. Your contractions will begin gradually and build up to four every 10 minutes towards the end of the first stage of labour. Near the end of your first stage of labour you may enter what is called 'a period of transition' where you feel slightly out of control or incapable of going any further with your labour. Your midwife will do her best to reassure you at this stage and support you through it.

The second stage of labour starts when your cervix is fully dilated and is completed with the birth of your baby. The second stage of labour is shorter than the first stage, usually between 1–3 hours. By now your cervix has dilated enough for your baby to pass through without causing any damage, and when the head has moved low enough you will begin feeling urges to push. This stage may make you feel quite shaky, as your muscles will be tired from the first stage, but you will be surprised at the surge of energy you get with these contractions. You are much stronger than you realise. It may feel as if your bowels are moving, but don't worry about this (your midwife certainly will not be bothered in the slightest): this sensation is a reaction to the pressure of the baby's head on your back passage, and it is not uncommon to pass some stools during this stage of labour. Each time you have a contraction, the baby moves farther and farther down. As you bear down (push), your baby's head begins to appear. Between contractions it will recede a little, but will move further down with each push until, finally, your baby is born.

You will be encouraged to gather up your baby into your arms, and if you do not feel able to do this, the midwife or your birth partner will pass you your baby. It was probably hard work at some points but the reward in your arms makes it worth every second. Congratulations to you both – you have already done a most important parenting task, you are already the most special people in the universe to your baby, and long may you keep up the good work.

The third stage of labour begins after the birth of your baby and is completed with the delivery of the placenta. If all went well with your delivery and your blood loss is within normal limits, you can ask your midwife for a natural third stage. Another option is to have an injection to make your uterus clamp down, so that your placenta is sheared off the wall of your uterus and your midwife can gently pull it out of you. Once your placenta is delivered it is time for a warm shower or bath, food and cuddles with your new baby. If you are not able to have an early discharge home then some hospitals will allow you to pay for a private room so that your birth partner can stay with you both.

Assisted births

There are two types of instrumentally assisted vaginal birth techniques: the vacuum extraction method and the use of forceps, as well as a surgically assisted method of birth called a caesarean section. Obstetricians usually do these types of deliveries, although in a few hospitals in England there are some midwives who have been trained to perform these procedures.

Vacuum extraction (also referred to as a ventouse delivery)

This is used to assist the birthing of your baby by applying suction to your baby's head. If you need help birthing your baby vaginally, have done most of the work yourself and your baby is not distressed, this is the best method. The vacuum cup will be applied to your baby's head, the suction started and as you push the doctor will gently angle and pull on your baby's head at the same time. It should not cause any trauma to you as the cup and hose are soft, but your baby's head may have a large blister for several days afterwards. The paediatrician can prescribe some painkillers for your baby, if necessary. Occasionally you may develop a tear as your baby is delivered by ventouse. Depending on how deep your tear is your midwife or the doctor who did the delivery may put in some stitches to help the wound edges heal in alignment.

Forceps

These are used if you or your baby are physically distressed by your labour, and if the baby is at an appropriate depth in your birth canal for this method to be effective. For this procedure you will need an episiotomy (a cut to your perineum) to widen the area where the doctor will need room in order to insert the forceps and clamp them around either side of your baby's head.

There may be some damage to your vagina or rectum and you will need stitches to help close the area where you were cut. The operating theatre team will be on standby before the doctor begins a forceps delivery in case the baby's head does not come down and deliver. If this is the case then you will need an emergency caesarean section. Soon after your placenta has been delivered your cut will be stitched up.

Caesarean section

This is the third type of assisted birth and involves delivery of your baby through a cut in your abdomen. It is used when a vaginal delivery is not possible or there is an immediate danger to you or your baby during labour. Some women mistakenly believe that the most sensible and safe way to birth a baby is by pre-planned caesarean section. This is not correct, as labour is a natural state for a woman's body to be in at the end of pregnancy, and you will heal much faster from a natural birth than from a surgical birth. If a caesarean is required then you will need to have an epidural inserted or, for emergency procedures, you will need a general anaesthetic. Caesareans are somewhat more risky because they involve major surgery and some type of anaesthesia, and infections, bleeding and wound complications occur more frequently with caesarean births. However, if you have had a caesarean because your health or your baby's health was at risk, then the value of this operation far outweighs the risks.

Vaginal birth after caesarean (VBAC)

Until very recently, most healthcare professionals thought that once a woman had a caesarean birth, any future babies should be delivered by another caesarean. Now certain women are supported to deliver vaginally after a previous caesarean birth. This option is not appropriate for everyone, but you can and should consider discussing this with your obstetrician or midwife to see if it is the best option for you.

When do I need to choose between a VBAC and a planned caesarean?

It is sensible to have an idea of what you want to do early in the pregnancy, and I would recommend that you discuss your options with the consultant and/or midwife at your 30-week antenatal check. A number of things can happen during your pregnancy that may alter your final plans, so I suggest that you finalise your delivery choice at about 36 weeks.

Please remember that natural vaginal births are the normal way to have your baby and the least physically stressful.

After surgical or instrumental births (and occasionally with vaginal births) you may have to have stitches. Ask your midwife how to care for your stitches in order to help yourself heal and please keep in mind that sometimes, despite your best efforts, you may still get an infection in this area. If this is the case then your doctor will prescribe antibiotics to help you clear the infection.

No matter which way you birth your baby, please make sure that as soon as possible afterwards you try to relax and begin regaining your strength as you gaze adoringly at your baby, or, while you sleep, your birth partner can spend some time gazing adoringly at you and your baby.

⏱ Exercise shortcuts

Walking is good exercise, but only if you walk fast enough to increase your heart rate a bit above normal (otherwise it is simply a form of transport). Try swinging your arms to just above your waist while walking to raise your heart rate.

 ## Health fact

Massage can make you feel great after a long day. Gentle face, shoulder, back, arm or hand massages are acceptable in pregnancy, but make sure the oils you use are safe at your stage of pregnancy and avoid foot massages, as stimulating certain parts of your foot can start your labour off.

 ## Be money wise

Milk powder costs a fraction of the price of regular milk but has the same nutritional value, so add it to hot cereal, mashed potatoes, hot drinks, soups and casseroles instead of fresh milk. (This advice applies only to adults and to children of seven years or older. Infants up to one year old should only have breast or formula milk, and children between one and seven years of age must have whole milk.)

ADDITIONAL ADVICE

Work

You'll probably be physically able to work during your entire pregnancy, though you may find you are very sleepy in the first few months and that you tire easily in the last few weeks. Your job shouldn't allow you to be exposed to chemicals or radiation, which may be dangerous to your baby. If you use chemicals as part of your work then please contact your occupational health department or your GP for advice. Some physical activities, such as lifting, may become impossible because of the changes pregnancy causes. Try to arrange short rest periods when you can sit and put your feet up. Many employers will allow you to shorten your lunch break and use the rest of this time as small periods of rest throughout the day. If you have complications which are related to your pregnancy, you may be advised to begin your maternity leave early. Remember that you can discuss your job situation with your midwife, union or HR department.

Travel

Travel is usually no risk to you or your baby if you follow certain guidelines. You shouldn't plan to travel long distances away from home during the last four to six weeks of your pregnancy and you should restrict your travel earlier if you're having twins, or have any pregnancy-related complications. When you do travel a long distance, make sure you are able to get up and walk around at least every two hours to help keep your circulation and other bodily functions working well. If an emergency arises and you must travel during the last four to six weeks of your pregnancy, ask your maternity health care provider for advice. Pack your maternity notes in case you need maternity care while away. Also you may need a doctor's note if you plan to travel by plane, as not all insurance companies are happy for you to travel without a doctor's approval. Please advise them you are pregnant when buying your insurance, or tell them if you become pregnant after buying your insurance. If any problems arise during the trip, go to the nearest medical facility immediately and take your maternity notes with you.

Baths

Some women wonder if it's safe to have a bath while they're pregnant, especially during the last months. The main problem when bathing while heavily pregnant is that some women find it a struggle to get out afterwards. So, in those last couple of months you should bathe when there is someone who can help you in and out of the bath. This will lessen your chance of straining yourself, slipping or falling at a time when you're not as likely to be able to stop and support yourself. The bath water temperature should be warm instead of hot, and if you enjoy using bubble bath make sure it is safe for use in pregnancy – for example, you should avoid using products containing essential oil of rose because if the concentration is high enough then there is a risk of miscarriage.

Tampons, Mooncups and other internal sanitary devices

Since you'll be having more vaginal discharge than usual, you might wonder about using tampons, Mooncups and the like. You need to keep your vagina as free from irritation and bacteria as possible, so it is recommended you try using lightweight mini-pads instead while pregnant. Then you won't have to worry about accidentally introducing extra germs into the already sensitive natural balance of your vagina.

Thrush

Should you develop thrush, try using plain, natural bio-yogurt before opting for a chemical treatment. You should find the yogurt works effectively to clear the thrush within three days and should ease the irritation immediately. Make sure to let your midwife or GP know if you think you have thrush, but you can begin using the yogurt before you see or speak to them. If your discharge is green, dark yellow, brown or blood-stained you should put a maternity pad on and call your local maternity hospital straight away.

Seat belts

Seat belts protect you and your baby in important ways. It's best you wear both the shoulder and lap belts, if possible. Place your lap belt under your abdomen, across your hips and thighs. Most baby injuries during pregnancy relate directly to the seriousness of the mother's injuries, rather than to those caused by the seat belt itself.

Clothing

Comfort is essential in pregnancy clothing. Wear a supportive bra, because your breasts will be getting larger and heavier. You may find soft-cup bras more comfortable and it's worth booking a bra fitting in the last trimester of your pregnancy to make sure you know what size you should be wearing. If you plan to wear tights, buy maternity tights instead of knee-high stockings. Make sure you have days when you wear skirts without tights and try to wear cotton underwear as frequently as possible. Support tights may help your legs if they're feeling tired or if you suffer from varicose veins, and your GP can prescribe these for you. It is recommended that you wear shoes that are flat or very low-heeled, and you may need wider-fit shoes as your pregnancy progresses because the tendons in your feet spread wider, due to the relaxing effects of the hormone changes surging through your body. I recommend that you focus on comfort in all your maternity clothes and shoes; nowadays many high-street and online retailers have relatively inexpensive and fashionable maternity clothing. Pregnancy can be very glamorous (as long as you don't show anyone your support tights!).

Caring for yourself

In order to make the most of your expectations and grow a beautiful, healthy baby, you need to take extra special care of yourself. Pregnancy can bring you both great joy and stress. As your weight and body changes, you'll need to alter some of your habits and routines. You might not be able to do everything you want to do for a few months. Remember, taking good care of yourself is taking good care of your baby. Here are some guidelines for taking good care of yourself.

Caring for your breasts

You may notice a slight leakage of fluid (colostrum) from your nipples during pregnancy, and towards the end of your pregnancy you may secrete quite a bit more. When washing your breasts use warm water, but no soap, and dry them well. If you have inverted nipples or develop them as your breasts enlarge, consult with your midwife or GP about exercises and equipment which may help to draw out your nipples. Milk cups or breast shields worn in your bra during the last part of the pregnancy may also help inverted nipples, but be careful they do not put too much pressure on your delicate breast tissue. Many maternity hospitals have lactation specialist midwives who will be happy to meet with you or refer you to their colleagues in your local well-woman centres during your pregnancy or postnatal period. Make sure to get your breast size measured at least twice during your pregnancy by an expert fitter, as you can increase several sizes during this time and you need to have a properly fitted bra. Otherwise they will be popping out of an improperly fitted one in the most awkward and embarrassing places possible. Take that as a word to the wise from one who has lived through the delights of breast pads continually making an appearance in an excruciatingly embarrassing fashion, until I gave in and admitted my bra was perhaps just a tad too small to contain everything that had to be kept in the cups! Be aware that breast milk has the uncanny capability of being able to stain every type of fabric it comes into contact with.

Teeth

As discussed earlier, proper dental care is very important. This is available for free from the NHS for all pregnant women. Don't hesitate to see your dentist if dental problems happen during your pregnancy. Just make sure your dentist knows you are pregnant so the proper precautions can be used when taking X-rays or prescribing medications. Make sure you brush your teeth at least twice a day with a soft-bristle brush because doing this, along with using dental floss and maintaining a proper diet, can minimise dental problems during pregnancy. Swollen and bleeding gums are common problems for pregnant women, but you must not ignore any bleeding without first consulting your dentist for advice.

Immunisation

Talk with your GP about immunisations you think you might need, such as the seasonal flu vaccine which is now available for all pregnant women, the MMR vaccine which is available to all women after they have had their baby and any injections which may be required for foreign travel. Some booster shots like tetanus are OK during pregnancy but others are not. You do not want to be given live virus vaccines during your pregnancy, as these are potentially harmful to your developing unborn child. Ideally, you should be appropriately immunised with live vaccines before you are pregnant. This allows a certain amount of immunity to be passed on from you to your child without the harmful effects a live virus might cause during pregnancy. Breastfeeding also passes on some natural immunity to your baby.

Insecticides and household chemicals

You should avoid heavy or prolonged exposure to as many household chemicals as possible. If you have to use strong household cleaning products, make sure you wear gloves and work in well-ventilated areas. You should also avoid weedkillers, pesticides and insecticides, unless you plan to travel and your GP advises you to use an insecticide such as mosquito repellent. Consider stopping using aerosol sprays and use mechanical pump sprayers or roller applicators instead, and avoid getting your hair dyed when pregnant. If you are painting your new nursery, be sure to use emulsion paint and work with the windows wide open, or preferably ask someone else to do the painting for you. Although oil-based paint and organic solvents like turpentine and lacquer have not been proven to be harmful, they do produce strong fumes that you should probably avoid.

Saunas, hot tubs and various therapies at your gym or spa

You can harm your baby if you raise the temperature of his/her environment over 38 degrees for prolonged periods of time, so it is best to avoid saunas, hot tubs and very hot baths while you're pregnant. If you need to soak your aching feet in very hot water that's fine, but avoid plunging in all the way. Reflexology with a qualified practitioner is fine as long as they are trained to treat pregnant women: otherwise there is a risk your labour could be started off. Some hospitals use reflexologists as a first resort to induce your labour when you are overdue before trying the chemical forms of induction.

Sex

The best rule here is that if it feels good and your pregnancy is uncomplicated, then go ahead and do it, in any position and as often as you wish. If you have a history of miscarriages, pregnancy-related vaginal bleeding or other complications then it is advisable that you don't have sex, and this will have been discussed with you at the time of identifying your particular pregnancy-related complication. Otherwise, there's absolutely no reason to interrupt your normal sex life. Orgasms will not start labour, cause bleeding or other problems during a normal pregnancy. Many partners are afraid that having sex will hurt the baby, but please try not to worry about this. Your baby is so well protected by fluid, muscle and bone that your movements are not going to bother him or her one little bit.

Useful things to have in your birth bag

- CDs, or MP3 player with your favourite and/or calming music saved onto a playlist

- Dried fruit, chewing gum or a few sweets, lip balm, non-fizzy soft drinks

- Pyjamas and whatever you plan to wear during labour

- Soap/shower gel, a flannel, towel, toothbrush and toothpaste

- Deodorant and other toiletries you use every day

- A toiletry kit for your birth partner

- Camera and/or mobile phone and charger

- Maternity pads (lots of them!), maternity/breastfeeding bra

- Something to tie or clip back your hair with, hairbrush

- A paper, hand-held fan

- Underpants (cotton, paper or a mix of the two – whichever you use, buy a larger size for comfort!), socks, a dressing gown and change of clothes

- A pillow of your own that you don't mind getting stained (hospital ones make crackling sounds because of the protective coating)

- Nappies, blanket and clothes for your baby

- Birth or labour plan/wish list

- A small amount of money, including some coins

- Any medication that you need to take every day

- Magazine for early labour

- TENS machine and a spare battery

- Maternity notes.

THE POSTNATAL MAP

Whether this is your first baby or your sixth, the thrill of seeing your new baby for the first time is finally here – a wonderful chance to bring about positive change in this world. All those months of expectation have come to life in one tiny baby; your own miracle. However, in the days and weeks to come it is important to also tell yourself that it is okay to feel tired and overwhelmed too.

Plan ahead

Most people with full-time jobs pre-parenthood are skilled in the art of time management, and this skill will come in handy when you have a new baby, especially during the first two or three months after you bring your baby home. You know that you're going to be tired, so if possible, plan to have some help during those first two months. But remember to make one point clear before friends or relatives arrive: you are taking care of the baby; they are taking care of the other essential chores that need doing, and not the other way around. If no one is close by to help, ask your midwife about home-visiting programmes and local postnatal support agencies, such as doulas and maternity nurses.

Plan to have your baby's clothes, nappies and bedding ready each day. Think of friends who have had babies in the last five years. Chances are they still have plenty of wearable and useable items that their children have outgrown. Babies have no concept of fashion trends, so why waste money on new clothes for them when there are plenty of good-quality second-hand items available?

Getting to know your baby

During your pregnancy you may have formed expectations about the gender and appearance of your baby. It may be difficult to reconcile these expectations with reality. It may also take a while for you and your family to get to know your new baby. Every baby is unique, and every parent's relationship with his or her baby is also unique. The first few days and weeks of your baby's life can be a marvellous adventure as you enjoy being a parent. However, when you are in pain and already sleep-deprived, it can be a struggle to form an immediate, deep bond with a demanding infant when you are also trying to cope with the demands of life as a new parent. I know of people (both mothers and fathers) who took up to two years to feel that they had bonded with their child. If you are having difficulty developing a bonded relationship with your baby, let your midwife, GP or health visitor know, as they can offer support and words of comfort in these situations.

Your own changes don't stop with the birth

Now that your months of great expectations have taken the form of a baby, you can expect more physical and mental changes in yourself during the weeks following the birth, much like those you experienced in early pregnancy. You'll be sore from the delivery, probably a little weak from overexertion of your muscles and quite tired.

Your hormone levels will return to normal and, in the process, your moods may swing much the same as in the beginning of pregnancy. Don't let these feelings frighten you because they will improve slowly over the next few weeks. You may experience some mild depression, commonly referred to as 'the baby blues', which shouldn't last more than a few days. However, postnatal depression is a serious condition that is different from baby blues. This can be more intense and overwhelming and will last longer. Any questions or concerns should be discussed with your midwife, GP or health visitor. They will be happy to advise you about support you may require in this period of your life, as well as ensuring you have medication, if it is needed.

You will have a bloody vaginal discharge for a while as the lining of your uterus sheds completely and your uterus will continue contracting as it returns to nearly its original size. Expect abdominal cramps for a few days after birth, especially if this is your second or third baby. These cramps may happen more often during breastfeeding, since breastfeeding causes the uterus to contract more noticeably. Your normal periods may not start again for several months if you are breastfeeding, but you may still become pregnant during this time if you don't use effective methods of contraception.

As discussed earlier, take all the help that is offered. Your most important job is to care for your baby and yourself. The vacuum cleaner won't mind if someone else uses it, or if it doesn't get used at all for a while. Try to avoid overexerting yourself in the first few weeks. Keep everything you need for your baby close to hand and let someone else get the shopping and do other chores for you for the first few days. Eventually, you will feel your strength and energy returning, especially if you challenge yourself to do a bit more each day to build up your strength. I think it is important to warn you that your stomach isn't instantly going to be flat again. Don't expect to leave the hospital and be back to your pre-pregnant size. It took nine months to get to that pre-birth size, so allow it the same amount of time to return to normal, but remember that you will now have a 'new normal', which will be slightly different from pre-pregnancy.

Gradually increase the amount of exercise you do. Begin with getting into a routine of doing your pelvic floor exercises, then start enjoying short, slow walks with your baby, and work your way up to speed walking with the buggy or pushchair, enjoy a mum-and-baby exercise class and, when you feel ready, take time out for yourself so you can indulge in a swim, a run or an exercise session at your local gym or community centre.

Pain relief and medications

If you are on regular medication of any kind, then make sure your GP reviews your medication so that you are taking the best one for this period of your life. This is particularly important if you are breastfeeding. Don't forget the healing power of gentle massage and the soothing properties of warm water. Take your baby into the bath with you; there is nothing stopping you from combining a feed with a chance for you to have a lovely long soak in warm (not hot) water. Make sure to keep a cloth over your baby's back or warm water part way up your baby's body so that he or she doesn't get chilled while feeding. Also have someone else nearby to make sure you don't fall asleep, and to take your baby from you when you are ready to get out.

Breastfeeding

Make sure that you get all the advice you can about learning how to tell if your baby is properly attached to the breast while feeding. This will help to ensure that feeding is comfortable for you, and that your baby gets all the food he or she needs. (From now on in this chapter, I'll alternate between 'he' and 'she' to refer to your baby.)

Sit or lie in a comfortable position. Hold your baby close to you, preferably skin to skin, without lots of blankets or clothing between you. Ensure that your baby is positioned so that his face and chest are facing the same way, with no twisting of the neck. Hold your baby so that you are supporting his back and shoulders, but make sure that you are not touching the back of his head, because your baby will need to be able to tip his head back. If you support your baby's back and shoulders then his head will still be well controlled. Your baby's nose should be opposite your nipple. Wait for your baby to open his mouth really wide. At this point bring his mouth swiftly towards your breast, making sure that his chin touches your breast first. When your baby is attached and sucking you can check to see if the attachment is good. His mouth should still appear to be wide open, and his bottom lip should be curled under itself. There should be more of your areola (the darker-coloured skin around your nipple) visible above your baby's top lip than below his bottom lip. Your baby's chin should be pushed into your breast and his cheeks should look full and rounded. The feed should feel comfortable, and you should have a sensation that your baby is sucking and swallowing, usually with one or two sucks to each swallow.

If you feel that your baby is not showing these signs of good attachment then it is advisable to reposition and reattach your baby to the breast. Release your nipple by inserting your little finger between your breast and your baby's mouth to break the seal, and then repeat the steps above. Your baby should relax into the feed, and it is very important to let him continue feeding for as long as he wishes, because the most fat-rich milk is at the end of the feed. When your baby has had enough milk he will detach from the breast without any effort on your part. It is important to keep your baby with you, so that you know when he wants to feed. He will show you his feeding cues by becoming more alert, sticking out his tongue, mouthing, turning his head to one side or making noises. It is best to try to feed him before he reaches the stage of crying.

Breastfeeding has many health benefits for both mothers and babies, both immediately and throughout their whole lives. Sometimes it may seem like hard work at first, but give it a couple of weeks and you will begin to realise the advantages of this method. When you are breastfeeding you can do nothing but rest yourself. There is no messing about with preparing feeds in bottles, saving you time and effort, and with the release of breast milk may come some 'feel good' hormones. To help you all bond as a family, try feeding your baby in bed, cradled between the two of you. Your partner can watch to make sure you don't fall asleep and help you by putting the baby in the cot after you have finished feeding, and by doing the nappy change if necessary.

Contrary to popular rumour, partners do like to help with the new baby! However, it is important to mention that although your breast milk is the best food for your baby, it is not always the best option for you. Some women cannot breastfeed for physical or psychological reasons, and this should not be viewed as a failure, but instead as an informed choice as to what is best for you and your baby.

Discomfort related to breastfeeding

If you find your breasts are uncomfortably engorged with milk at any stage then it is important to check that your baby is positioned and attached to your breast correctly. The most effective way of relieving engorgement is to feed your baby frequently, making sure that you respond to his cues and not leaving long gaps between feeds. You could hand-express a little milk to make yourself more comfortable, and doing this before a feed can also help to make it easier for your baby to attach when your breasts are very firm. Some women find that placing cooled Savoy cabbage leaves or flannels on their breasts may help with the discomfort, but feeding or hand-expressing are the best ways to resolve the problem.

Some women end up with cracked nipples during the first few weeks of breastfeeding. The best cure for this is understanding how to latch and unlatch your baby properly. If you are not sure then please read the section above or contact your midwife or local maternity unit for support. Your midwife may also recommend that you join a breastfeeding support group. I went to one of these each week for months simply because I enjoyed being in the company of other breastfeeding mums! You may also find that rubbing in leftover breast milk after a feed and allowing your nipples to air-dry will speed the healing process. If you feel they are too sore to latch your baby comfortably, then expressing a small amount before latching your baby on should help to dull the latching sensation.

Formula feeding

If you choose not to breastfeed or if you decide to change to bottle-feeding your baby, then you will discover that there is a wide variety of formulas on offer as well as the option of offering expressed breast milk by bottle. Most infant feed formulas do their best to chemically mimic the qualities of breast milk, but they all vary from each other slightly. You may need to try a few before you find the one that suits your baby best. All the equipment used to make up formula feeds and to feed the formula to your baby must be sterilised. This includes if you choose to feed your baby breast milk from a bottle. There are different methods you can use to do this, including sterilising solution and microwavable sterilising kits. Whichever method you choose, please ensure you follow the directions for that method. The same goes for preparing formula feeds – prepare them exactly according to the instructions on the packet and feed them to your baby as frequently as instructed on the packet for your baby's weight and age.

Don't forget that help is available both before and after birth in regards to feeding your baby (whether you are breast- or bottle-feeding), so ask your midwife for help if you need it.

Resuming lovemaking after giving birth

Your normal periods may not start again for several months if you are breastfeeding, but you can still get pregnant again as early as 21 days after birth, so make sure you use contraception. You may be thinking that there is no way you could possibly want to make love so soon after giving birth, especially with a demanding baby to care for, but hormones are funny things. So unless you want your children very close in age, I strongly recommend that you make sure you use contraception and that it is effective.

Contraception choices

Barrier methods

These are condoms (both male and female versions) and the diaphragm. If you used a diaphragm before pregnancy, then you need to ask your GP to check to make sure your old one still fits properly before you begin using it again after you have had your baby. Your GP will not be able to check this until at least six weeks after you have had your baby because your cervix is still closing and shrinking up to this point. Properly applied condoms are up to 98 per cent effective at preventing conception and properly fitted diaphragms used with a spermicide are up to 96 per cent effective.

Oral contraceptive pill

Your GP will likely recommended the progesterone-only pill if you wish to use this method in the postnatal period, because it is safe with breastfeeding. It's also safe if you have a pregnancy-related condition that your body is still recovering from, such as high blood pressure. If the pill is taken within the same time frame each day then it is up to 99 per cent effective, but it does not provide protection against sexually transmitted infections. If you have a stomach virus causing you to vomit or have diarrhoea, then you must use another form of contraception for as long as your GP, sexual health nurse or chemist advises.

Long-acting reversible contraceptive

These are contraceptive injections, implants or devices such as the hormonal coil. You will not be able to have a coil fitted until at least four weeks after giving birth, but you may be able to have the injection or implant earlier than this. These methods provide high protection against conception but will not protect you against sexually transmitted infections.

Emergency contraception

This works by preventing ovulation, fertilisation of an egg or implantation of a fertilised egg in your uterus on a one-off basis. Emergency contraception is not suitable to be used as a regular form of contraception because – as the name implies – it is designed for emergency use only. Should you need to use this form of contraception then it is available free from all contraception clinics and pharmacies, but you may be charged if you need to get it from a pharmacy.

Your midwife, health visitor, sexual health nurse or GP can advise you as to what contraception will work best for you as an individual. If you would like to consider your options in more detail first then you can visit the *My Mini Midwife* section on my website to find a link to the most up-to-date information: **www.djkirkby.co.uk/my-mini-midwife**.

Newborn bloodspot screening

Between day five to day eight of your baby's life, you will be offered several routine blood tests for your baby, which can all be done from blood collected onto a piece of special card from one heel prick. This series of blood tests checks your baby for congenital hypothyroidism (underactive thyroid), cystic fibrosis (abnormally thick mucus and altered levels of certain digestive enzymes), phenylketonuria (allergy to the protein phenalynine), and MCADD (a metabolic disorder). You should receive a leaflet about this from your midwife during your pregnancy, but if you have misplaced it or if you want more details about any of the screening and diagnostic tests in this book, please visit **www.djkirkby.co.uk/my-mini-midwife**, where you will find links to the most-up-to-date leaflets available.

Newborn hearing screening

This is a non-invasive test that is usually done on babies within the first few days of life to test for hearing problems. If there are any concerns, then your baby will be referred for further testing. Again, you can find links to up-to-date information about this at **www.djkirkby.co.uk/my-mini-midwife**, if you need it.

Newborn and infant physical examination

The newborn part of this test is done within the first 72 hours after birth, and the infant part of this test is done by the time your baby has reached eight weeks of age. It is a top-to-toe physical examination of your baby's body which checks to make sure things (such as testicles) are where they should be and things like the heart, lungs, eyes and so on are working as expected. For more details about any of the screening and diagnostic tests in this book, please visit **www.djkirkby.co.uk/my-mini-midwife** for links to the most up-to-date leaflets available.

Monitoring for signs of infection in your baby

You will soon begin to recognise what your baby's normal behaviours are, but even before that happens you will be able to make sure your baby is well if she is waking to feed regularly without prompting from you.

Signs of infection can include any of the following signs, and you should seek urgent advice from your GP, midwife or health visitor if you spot any of them:

- Your baby's skin and whites of eyes turn yellow (a tinge of yellow is often perfectly normal, but ask your midwife or GP to check this for you).

- Your baby's skin develops a rash – some rashes are normal, but ask your midwife, health visitor or GP to check the rash (they may ask you to describe it over the phone).

- Your baby is hotter or colder than usual (both can be signs of infection). If this happens, then strip your baby down to her nappy and place her in direct contact with your bare skin (covering any of her bare skin with a blanket). Call your midwife, GP or health visitor for further advice while you are having this skin-to-skin contact.

- Your baby is unexplainably irritable over a longer period than the usual pre-sleep or pre-feed grumpiness, or your baby seems to be shivering.

- Your baby vomits in between feeds and the fluid is yellow, green or brown (rather than the usual milky-coloured possets your baby may do shortly after feeds).

- Your baby makes 'grunting' or gasping sounds while breathing, or you can see the nostrils flaring with each breath.

I remember one big sister refusing to look in the cot when she came to meet her new baby brother for the first time, because she thought he sounded like a piglet. She had asked for a brother, not a piglet, and was most indignant that her parents had got it so wrong. Her brother had been born by emergency caesarean section and was a bit mucusy because he was trying to clear the fluid from his chest that would have drained during the course of a vaginal birth. His big sister interpreted this grunty breathing as the same sounds as a piglet might make. Babies can also sound grunty if they are unwell, though, so it is wise to let your maternity care giver know if you think your baby is making these sounds, or if you notice your baby's nostrils flaring.

Health fact

The nutritional benefits from quinoa, including the fact that it is a complete protein (unlike other grains), gluten free and high in calcium (useful for vegans), have led to it earning its 'super food' nickname, and it's great for bulking out a lunchtime salad.

Be money wise

Use leftover chilli or ratatouille as an inexpensive alternative to pasta sauces. You can also stretch it further by adding another tin of chopped tomatoes. If you have the space in your freezer, then in the final months of your pregnancy make meals and freeze them ready for use while you are busy getting into a routine of parenting your new baby.

FREQUENTLY ASKED QUESTIONS

How do I know if I am pregnant?

You will miss a period, or your periods will become lighter. Your nipples or breasts may become very tender. The best way to know for sure if you are pregnant or not is to take a pregnancy test, and if you are uncertain what the test result is then take it with you to your GP to discuss it further.

Can I drink alcohol when I am pregnant?

Research has proven that alcohol is harmful to your baby while pregnant or breastfeeding. What we don't know yet is exactly how much, and at what point during your pregnancy. It is thought that in the majority of pregnancies it should be safe to drink one or two units per week, but the only way to be sure that alcohol will not harm your baby is to not drink any alcohol during pregnancy.

Why didn't my baby come on the due date I was given?

Many women have different-length menstrual cycles and this, along with other things, can affect the length of their pregnancies by days or even weeks. It is best to think of your due date as a 'due week', but also be aware that your baby is full term anytime from 37 weeks onwards and some babies are not ready to be born before the pregnancy has lasted 42 weeks.

How much blood will I lose after the baby?

You will lose more blood than you do during a normal period for the first few days after you give birth and you will need to wear special maternity pads during this time which are more absorbent and made with fewer chemicals than most non-maternity sanitary pads. After the first few days your blood loss should slow down to an amount similar to when you have your period and ease off gradually from then. Your loss will be bright red at first, then turn pink, then brown and eventually just creamy or clear; it shouldn't smell any different from a normal period at any time. If it does, then please tell your midwife, GP or health visitor.

Do I really need to buy maternity pads or can I bring in my pre-pregnancy menstrual pads?

See the blood-loss answer above.

I only used tampons before pregnancy, so can I use those instead of pads after I have had my baby?

Tampons, Mooncups and other internal menstrual devices should not be used until after you have had your 6–8-week postnatal check by your GP.

When can we go home from hospital?

This will depend on what kind of a labour and birth you had and how well you and the baby are afterwards. Some women go home as early as just a few hours after birth, while others may need to stay in for a few days. Alternatively, women who had a home birth may need to be admitted to hospital if they have complications after their birth.

Can my birth partner stay in hospital with my baby and me?

Due to the fact that birthing rooms are in high demand and postnatal rooms are usually occupied by more than one woman, birth partners staying in hospital for more than a few hours after birth is only considered acceptable in exceptional circumstances.

Do I have to have my baby in hospital?

If all is well with you and your baby during your pregnancy and labour, then a home birth should be an option for you. However, this is also dependent on other factors, such as the conditions and location you live in, staffing levels during the time you are in labour and the clinical opinion of the midwife caring for you at the time. When you discuss your choice of place of birth with your midwife she will be able to give you some idea of how likely it is that you will be able to birth at home, if this is your wish. Regardless of place of birth, you may wish to think through a birth plan, and the NHS Choices website offers ready-made templates which you can print off and complete, ready to share with the midwife caring for you in labour. These can be found by going to the NHS Choices website (www.nhs.uk) and typing 'birth plan' into the search bar.

Why does my baby wake up to feed so often at night?

A healthy baby will wake to feed every few hours, and this includes throughout the night. This is because a baby's stomach is tiny for the first few months of life and therefore he needs to feed little and often to stay healthy and well hydrated. Many babies are sleeping through the night by the time they are a year old.

How do I know if my baby has had enough to eat?

It is easy to tell if a breastfed baby has had enough to eat as she will usually spontaneously stop feeding when she is full.

See the breastfeeding section in 'The Postnatal Map' chapter (page 124) for further details on this. If you are feeding your baby with formula milk then you will need to be guided by the instructions on the packaging, which will give you details of how much formula a baby should have based on age and weight. A baby who has had enough food and has been winded will be content after a feed. It is normal for babies to want to eat little and often in the first few months of life as their tummies are very tiny. Demand feeding your baby (supplying breast milk when your baby wants it) is simple and safe, as your body will adapt to produce the type of milk your baby requires (for example, sometimes watery, rather than filling, milk), but the same process is a bit more complicated with formula feeding, as you must be careful not to give more formula than the packaging advises.

How often do I bathe my baby?

This depends on the individual baby and the age. Newborns do not need bathing for the first few days, and this time gives them a chance to adjust to their new environment without subjecting them to chemicals such as soap. Newborns and older babies do need to have their nappy area cleansed with warm water and cotton wool (or a soft flannel) and dried with each nappy change. They also need to have their face and any area where fluids such as milk, post-feed possets and saliva will run (such as folds of skin on neck, under arms and behind ears) wiped clean with warm water and cotton wool or a soft flannel and dried at least twice a day.

How do I establish a routine and at what age?

This is a very difficult question to answer because all babies and families are different. Babies are born with individual feeding and sleeping routines that they need to follow for at least the first month until they are fully adapted to their new environment. You can, however, introduce regular routines, such as going for walks and bathing time, after the first week or so, once you have begun to adjust to life with the newest member of your family. For example, you may wish to play soothing music and show your baby black-and-white picture books (because it is easier for him to see these than colours) mid-morning, go for a walk each day with your baby in a sling or pram around mid-afternoon and bathe your baby every evening at the same time. You can gradually build your routines to cover regular activities such as getting showered or bathed, and getting you and baby dressed and fed each morning. All of these things will help you practise getting ready to leave the house by a certain time each day in readiness for going back to work, if this is something you will need to do in the future. These are just examples and you should combine whatever activities and timings suit you, your baby and your lifestyle.

What do I do if my baby cries?

It will take you a few weeks to work out that your baby cries in a different way to ask for or to complain about different things. Until you decipher the cry code you will need to run through a checklist of the following problems that may be troubling your baby:

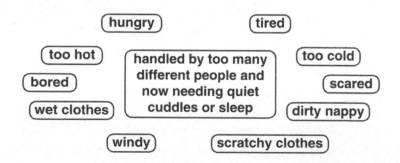

You will soon add things to this list that affect your baby as an individual.

Some people have a special knack for calming even the most outraged of babies. I used to work with someone who would cradle the crying baby, smoothing his back for a while before shifting him higher up on her shoulder until her mouth was level with his ear. She would then make a strange, low-pitched moaning sound. The baby would quieten almost immediately and within a minute would have relaxed completely, still alert but calm and listening to the noise my colleague was making, and before too much longer he would be fast asleep. I watched her many times and her technique never failed. I have tried to mimic this skill many times since, with varying success, and would recommend it to anyone wishing to have a go at it.

Do I swaddle?

The answer to this again depends on your baby's individual personality: some babies enjoy being swaddled, whilst others dislike it. The only way you will find out is to try it.

- Spread a cotton sheet out on a flat and dry surface.

- Make sure your baby is dressed in no more than a vest and Babygro or similar (two thin layers of clothing, not including the nappy). Lay your baby on her back on the sheet, with her neck resting against the fold at the top of the sheet.

- Wrap the top left-hand corner of the sheet across your baby's body and tuck it under her left arm.

- Bring the bottom left-hand corner over her feet, and then wrap the right corner around her back, leaving only her head and neck exposed.

- Allow enough room for your baby to move her hips and knees freely, so she can move her knees up and outwards.

- Pay attention to the temperature of your baby to ensure she doesn't get too hot while being swaddled; it is better for your baby to be on the cooler side than too warm. Babies like their internal temperature to be between 36.5 and 37.2 degrees Celsius – exactly where your baby prefers to be in this range will be different to other babies' preferences.

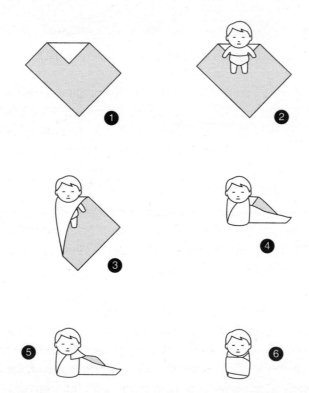

How many outfits do I need in the beginning?

You will need to change your baby each time their clothing gets wet, which usually happens when they bring up excess milk after a feed, or with very wet or dirty nappies. If you are planning a hospital birth, then you need to pack several sleep suits and baby vests, as well as a couple of baby blankets, which should be enough to last you a day or two. If you are not planning to stay in hospital for more than a few hours after the birth, then a couple of changes of clothing and one baby blanket should be adequate for your baby's needs. Some people like their babies to wear different clothes for day wear and sleep wear, so pack according to your preferences, and you may also wish to pack a 'going-home outfit' for your baby. If you end up staying in hospital longer than planned, then you can ask someone to bring in extra clothing for you and your baby.

If you are planning to birth at home you should still have a case packed for you and your baby in case your midwife decides you need to transfer to hospital during labour (or just after delivery), should there be any complications during this period of time.

How are surrogacies arranged?

There are agencies specialising in offering surrogacy support and these can be found by searching for 'surrogacy' on the Internet. I recommend that you choose one that operates as a not-for-profit support organisation.

Why choose surrogacy over adoption?

You may decide to choose surrogacy over adoption because this option will allow the baby to carry genetic material from one parent (in the form of sperm donation, which is also referred to as 'traditional' surrogacy) or both parents (in the form of *in vitro* fertilisation, where sperm is used to fertilise an egg outside the body, which is then implanted in the uterus; this is also called gestational surrogacy).

ACKNOWLEDGEMENTS

Huge thanks to everyone on Facebook and Twitter who asked me questions for the FAQ section in *My Mini Midwife*.

Thank you to Dr Catherine Angell for her advice with the wording of the breastfeeding section.

Thank you to Denise Spendlove (a diabetic specialist midwife) for her advice with the wording of the diabetes section.

Grateful thanks to the editors who worked on *My Mini Midwife* – Claire Plimmer, Abbie Headon, Anna Martin and Justine Gore-Smith.

GLOSSARY

A

Abdominal pain – pain in the area below the belly button
Amniocentesis – a diagnostic test
Areola – the darker tissue around your nipple

B

Braxton Hicks contractions – practice contractions that do not dilate the cervix

C

Caesarean section – operative delivery of your baby
Cannula – a thin tube inserted into your body (often into a vein) through which fluids or medication are injected
Cervix – the opening to your womb
Chorionic villus sampling (CVS) – a diagnostic test
Colostrum – the fluid produced by your breasts in late pregnancy until milk is made a couple of days after birth

Conception – the beginning of your pregnancy
Constipation – difficulty having bowel movements
Contractions – tightening of your uterus
Cramps – mild to moderate pain in your abdomen
Cravings – unexpectedly strong urges for a specific food

D

Diagnostic testing – a test that gives a definite 'yes' or 'no' answer, like amniocentesis or chorionic villus sampling
Dilating – increasing the opening of the cervix, usually during labour
Down's Syndrome – a chromosomal disorder, one of the three trisomies

E

Early-pregnancy bleeding – blood loss from the vagina before 12 weeks of pregnancy
Early labour – the beginning of labour, when contractions are still irregular and not very painful
Edward's Syndrome – a chromosomal disorder, one of the three trisomies
Engagement – when the presenting part of your baby descends into the opening of your pelvis
Engorgement – when your breasts are uncomfortably full of milk
Entonox – a short-acting, breathable form of pain relief
Epidural – a long-lasting, invasive form of pain relief
Established labour – when contractions are regular and long-lasting

F

False labour – a term used to refer to labour that is not yet established

First trimester combined screening – non-diagnostic testing, usually done before 12 weeks of pregnancy

Fluid retention – swelling during pregnancy

Forceps – special tongs used to grip onto parts of your or your baby's body

Fundus – the top of the uterus

G

Genetic screening – may be done during the first trimester combined screening, amniocentesis and CVS

Group B streptococcus (GBS) – a rare infection that can cause damage to babies

H

Haemorrhoids – piles, varicose veins in the vulval or rectal area

Headaches – these are common in the early stages of pregnancy, but can be a symptom of raised blood pressure later on in pregnancy

Heartburn – common during pregnancy, especially in the latter stages

Herbal tea – not all herbal teas are safe in pregnancy

High blood pressure – can cause headaches and other problems in pregnancy

Hormone levels – these can be measured as part of pregnancy investigations, and are responsible for emotional mood swings

Hydrotherapy – deep, warm water baths in special pools can provide pain relief during labour

Hypnosis – used by some women during labour as a form of pain relief

I

Immunisations – offered to women during pregnancy, after birth and to babies and infants

Induction of labour – used to try and start labour if necessary

Infectious diseases – routine screening during pregnancy offered to all women

Insomnia – changes to sleep patterns are common during pregnancy, including periods of being awake at night

L

Labour – the lead-up to childbirth

Late-pregnancy bleeding – bleeding in the third trimester

Libido – sex drive

M

Massage – used by some women as a form of pain relief in labour

Medication – take only on medical advice during pregnancy and while breastfeeding

Monitoring in labour – this will occur in various forms and is used to asses your and your baby's wellbeing

Mood swings – very common during pregnancy

'Morning' sickness – nausea and vomiting during pregnancy that can occur any time of the day

N

Nausea – feeling sick
NICE – National Institute for Health and Care Excellence
NMC Nursing and Midwifery Council
Nosebleeds – can occur during pregnancy
Nuchal scan – a scan which measures your baby's nuchal fold thickness between 11 and 14 weeks as a predictor of risk for certain conditions

P

Pain relief – can be internal or external, short-term or long-lasting
Patau's Syndrome – a chromosomal disorder, one of the three trisomies
PHE – Public Health England
Pelvic pressure – feeling pressure in your pelvis during pregnancy and labour
Perineum – a hammock-like layered structure of muscles that stretch from your pubic bone down around your vagina and up past your anus
Pessary – medicine in a large tablet shape that is inserted into the vagina or rectum
Pet litter – should not be changed unless wearing gloves during pregnancy
Pethidine – an injected, long-lasting form of pain relief
Pica – craving non-nutritional substances such as ice or coal during pregnancy
Piles (see under Haemorrhoids)
Placental abruption – when the placenta separates partially or completely from the uterine wall during pregnancy or in labour before the baby is delivered

Placenta praevia – when your placenta partially or completely covers your cervix

Postnatal – the first month after birth

Pre-conception – the time before you begin trying to get pregnant

Pre-eclampsia – a pregnancy disorder linked to high blood pressure.

Pregnancy – from conception until the birth of your baby

Premature labour – labour before 37 weeks of pregnancy

Prescription medications – medicine prescribed by a doctor or midwife

Prolonged ruptured membranes – when your waters break but labour does not begin within 12–72 hours (the time frame varies between hospitals)

R

RCOG – Royal College of Obstetricians and Gynaecologists

RCM – Royal College of Midwives

Recreational drugs – medicines not prescribed by a doctor or midwife that alter your perception

Real labour – when your contractions are regular, long-lasting and cause your cervix to dilate

'Red-hot pokers' – shooting pains felt in the vagina during the later stages of pregnancy

Relaxin – a hormone that helps your body stretch to accommodate your growing baby

Round ligament pain – stretching or stitch-type pain usually felt during the first 12 weeks of pregnancy

Rupture of membranes – when your waters break

S

Screening – investigations done during pregnancy to monitor your and your baby's health

Sperm count – this varies depending on the age and health of the man and the type of underwear worn

Stretch marks – visible changes in the elasticity of your skin during pregnancy to accommodate your growing baby

Swelling – can occur at any stage of pregnancy

T

TENS – electronic pain relief

Tiredness – common at the beginning and end stages of pregnancy

Trans-abdominal CVS – diagnostic testing in early pregnancy

Trans-cervical CVS – diagnostic testing in early pregnancy

U

Ultrasound screening/scan – imaging of your baby during pregnancy to look for structural defects

Uncomfortable breathing – should always be checked out by a doctor or midwife

V

Vacuum extraction – an instrumental delivery of your baby

Vaginal birth – non-operative delivery of your baby

Vaginal birth after caesarean (VBAC) – a non-operative birth after having had an operative delivery the time before

Vaginal discharge – the amount will vary throughout your pregnancy but should never be red, brown or green

Varicose veins – see piles and haemorrhoids

Vulva – the area that includes the labia and the muscles around your vagina

W

Weight – should be within a normal healthy range before getting pregnant for the best pregnancy health outcomes for you and your baby

LINKS TO ADDITIONAL INFORMATION

At **www.djkirkby.co.uk/my-mini-midwife** you will find the dedicated page on my website where you can access links for up-to-date additional supporting information for all the screening and diagnostic tests and other topics discussed in *My Mini Midwife*.

NOTES

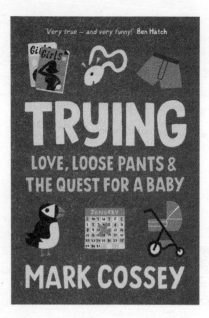

Trying
Love, Loose Pants and the Quest for a Baby

Mark Cossey

ISBN: 978-1-84953-398-0

Paperback

£8.99

'Here again, Mr Cossey?' asked the young Spanish embryologist, shooting me a welcoming smile as I followed him down the corridor. He had recognised me by sight and that wasn't good. I was now the one thing you don't want to be in a fertility clinic. A regular.

Martha wanted a baby. Mark wanted a baby. What's the worst that could happen?

In four years of baby-making boot camp, Mark and Martha face The Calendar, the anti-wank chair, hostile cervical mucus, IUI, IVF and the possibility of being childless. Through a combination of ignorance and outrage, Mark overcomes the challenges of ejaculating into a small jar, stabbing his wife, having his sperm turned pink and group sex with whales, and eventually sees his and Martha's ultimate dream come true – a family of their own.

It says a lot when you can call two years of sleepless nights a happy ending.

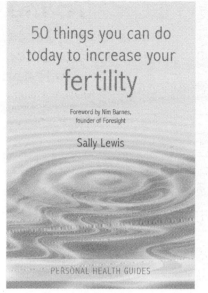

50 Things You Can Do Today to Increase Your Fertility

Sally Lewis

ISBN: 978-1-84953-119-1

Paperback

£6.99

In this easy-to-follow book, Sally explains how diet, weight, stress and many other factors affect fertility. She offers practical advice and a holistic approach to help you increase your fertility, including simple lifestyle changes and DIY complementary therapies. Find out 50 things you can do today including:

- Choose fertility-boosting foods and supplements
- Discover the best time for conception
- Understand the link between body, mind and fertility
- Find helpful organisations and products

'This book is well worth reading; it is full of valuable advice for all couples hoping to conceive'　　　　Nim Barnes, founder of Foresight

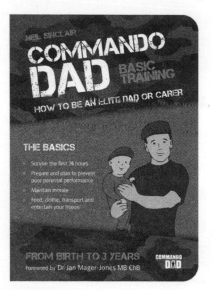

COMMANDO DAD
How to Be an Elite Dad or Carer

Neil Sinclair

ISBN: 978-1-84953-261-7

Paperback

£9.99

From Birth to 3 Years

In your hand is an indispensable training manual for new recruits to fatherhood. Written by ex-Commando and dad of three, Neil Sinclair, this manual will teach you, in no-nonsense terms, how to:

- Plan for your baby trooper's arrival
- Prepare nutritious food for yor unit
- Maintain morale and keep the troops entertained

And much, much more. Let training commence!

'One of the best parenting books I've ever read.'   Lorraine Kelly

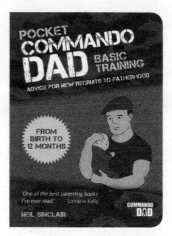

POCKET
COMMANDO
DAD
Advice for New Recruits to Fatherhood

Neil Sinclair

ISBN: 978-1-84953-555-7

Paperback

£7.99

From Birth to 12 Months

This pocket-sized, no-nonsense training manual for new dads will teach you how to:

- Prepare base camp for your baby trooper's arrival

- Survive the first 24 hours

- Establish feeding/sleeping routines

And much, much more. Let training commence!

'easy to understand and simple to digest… spot on'   THE GUARDIAN

'a revolutionary new parenting book'   GRAZIA